Competency in Combining Pharmacotherapy and Psychotherapy

Integrated and Split Treatment

Second Edition

T0176385

Competency in Combining Pharmacotherapy and Psychotherapy

Integrated and Split Treatment

Second Edition

Michelle B. Riba, M.D., M.S.
Richard Balon, M.D.
Laura Weiss Roberts, M.D., M.A.

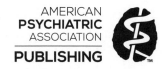

AMERICAN
PSYCHIATRIC
ASSOCIATION
PUBLISHING

If you wish to buy 50 or more copies of the same title, please go to www.appi.org/specialdiscounts for more information.

Copyright © 2018 American Psychiatric Association Publishing

ALL RIGHTS RESERVED

Second Edition

Manufactured in the United States of America on acid-free paper
21 20 19 18 17   5 4 3 2 1

American Psychiatric Association Publishing
1000 Wilson Boulevard
Arlington, VA 22209-3901
www.appi.org

Library of Congress Cataloging-in-Publication Data
Names: Riba, Michelle B., author. | Balon, Richard, author. | Roberts, Laura Weiss, 1960– author. | American Psychiatric Association, issuing body.
Title: Competency in combining pharmacotherapy and psychotherapy : integrated and split treatment / by Michelle B. Riba, Richard Balon, Laura Weiss Roberts.
Description: Second edition. | Arlington, Virginia : American Psychiatric Association Publishing, [2018] | Includes bibliographical references and index.
Identifiers: LCCN 2017043765 (print) | LCCN 2017044622 (ebook) | ISBN 9781615371808 (ebook) | ISBN 9781615370665 (pbk. : alk. paper)
Subjects: | MESH: Mental Disorders—therapy | Psychotherapy—methods | Drug Therapy—methods | Combined Modality Therapy—methods | Clinical Competence
Classification: LCC RC483 (ebook) | LCC RC483 (print) | NLM WM 140 | DDC 616.89/18--dc23
LC record available at https://lccn.loc.gov/2017043765

British Library Cataloguing in Publication Data
A CIP record is available from the British Library.

Contents

Preface

Millions of people each year live with a mental disorder that causes significant distress and disability. In economically established countries, the evidence-informed practice of combining pharmacotherapy and psychotherapy has become the most frequently used approach in caring for these people. Most clinicians endorse the combination of pharmacotherapy and psychotherapy as more efficacious and beneficial than each modality alone.

Combining medication and psychosocial treatments may seem like a simple additive process, but it is complicated and highly variable. Pharmacotherapy may be combined with brief therapy, cognitive-behavioral therapy, psychodynamic psychotherapy, supportive psychotherapy, or many other therapies. The combination of medication treatment and psychotherapy may be delivered by one person (integrated treatment) or by two or more persons (split/collaborative treatment) and may occur in the context of primary care or highly subspecialized psychiatric care.

Psychiatrists and psychiatric residents should demonstrate competency in combining and coordinating treatment modalities for the benefit of their patients. Learning how to approach and master integrated and split/collaborative care as a patient-centered therapeutic strategy is critically important. Because of the rapid transformation of clinical care models in new health systems, competence in integrated and split/collaborative care is vital for psychiatrists long established in the field and for psychiatrists early in their professional development.

This book is a basic text intended for residents, teaching faculty, and early-career psychiatrists. The text focuses on competency in combining pharmacotherapy and psychotherapy and also touches on advanced topics such as evaluation, monitoring, and supervision; best practices in terminating and transitioning patient care; and primary care access for mental health services in the context of integrated and split/collaborative care. The book has three main sections. The first deals with integrated treatment, the second focuses on split/collaborative care, and the third focuses on advanced topics.

For psychiatric educators, we note that the Accreditation Council for Graduate Medical Education (ACGME) has six main competencies: patient care and procedural skills, medical knowledge, practice-based learning and improvement, interpersonal and communication skills, professionalism, and systems-based practice (see table on opposite page). This book relates to all six. It should also be helpful for educators in relation to the recently revised Milestones (Holombe et al. 2016) of the ACGME and the recently introduced Core Entrustable Professional Activities of the Association of American Medical Colleges (2014). We direct the reader to the Appendix ("Review Questions on Competencies Related to Integrated and Split/Collaborative Care").

The aim of every psychiatrist is to lessen distress and enhance well-being in people living with mental health conditions by using the best evidence-derived methods of the field. It is no surprise that optimal care for many disorders will arise from the intentional combination of two or more of these methods. Learning when and how to put these combinations into practice is crucial work, helping patients to have healthier, more fulfilling lives through access to state-of-the-art clinical care.

The authors offer their sincere appreciation to Gabrielle Termuehlen and Katie Ryan for their many contributions to this text. Ms. Termuehlen provided editorial assistance in developing the second edition, and Ms. Ryan greatly helped with the background research included in the updated edition.

Richard Balon, M.D.
Michelle B. Riba, M.D., M.S.
Laura Weiss Roberts, M.D., M.A.

References

Association of American Medical Colleges: Core Entrustable Professional Activities for Entering Residency: Faculty and Learners' Guide. 2014. Available at: https://members.aamc.org/eweb/upload/Core%20EPA%20Faculty%20and%20Learner%20Guide.pdf. Accessed May 23, 2017.
Holombe ES, Edgar L, Hamstra S: The Milestones Guidebook, Version 2016. ACGME. Available at: http://www.acgme.org/Portals/0/MilestonesGuidebook.pdf. Accessed May 23, 2017.

Core competencies (in bold) and milestones related to integrated and split/collaborative care

Patient care and procedural skills

Psychiatric evaluation

Psychiatric formulation and differential diagnosis

Treatment planning

Psychotherapy

Somatic therapies

Medical knowledge

Psychotherapy

Somatic therapies

Practice-based learning and improvement

Formal practice-based quality improvement based on established and accepted methodologies

Interpersonal and communications skills

Relationship development, conflict management with patients, families, colleagues, and members of the health care team

Information sharing and record keeping

Professionalism

Compassion, integrity, respect for others, sensitivity to diverse patient population, adherence to ethical principles

Accountability to self, patients, colleagues, and the profession

Systems-based practice

Resource management

About the Authors

Michelle B. Riba, M.D., M.S., is Clinical Professor and Program Director of the Psychosomatic Medicine Fellowship; Associate Director of the University of Michigan Comprehensive Depression Center; and Director of the Psych-Oncology Program at the University of Michigan Comprehensive Cancer Center in Ann Arbor, Michigan.

Richard Balon, M.D., is Professor, Departments of Psychiatry and Behavioral Neurosciences and Anesthesiology; and Associate Chair for Education and Program Director at the Department of Psychiatry and Behavioral Neurosciences at Wayne State University School of Medicine in Detroit, Michigan.

Laura Weiss Roberts, M.D., M.A., is Katharine Dexter McCormick and Stanley McCormick Memorial Professor and Chair of the Department of Psychiatry and Behavioral Sciences at Stanford University School of Medicine in Stanford, California.

Introduction to Integrated and Split/Collaborative Treatment

1

Millions of individuals living with mental illness in the United States could, or do, greatly benefit from psychiatric care that addresses both biological and psychosocial considerations. For the past 30 years, psychiatric care for most mental disorders in the United States has been increasingly characterized by psychopharmacological treatment (Correll et al. 2011; Olfson et al. 2012, 2014) and evidence-based psychotherapies such as cognitive-behavioral therapy and interpersonal therapy, including collaborative care in primary care contexts (Katon and Unützer 2013; Raney 2015). For many psychiatrists in the United States, the provision of psychotherapy may not be as profitable as providing medication or other treatments alone. Nevertheless, evidence-based practice guidelines recommend that psychiatrists provide psychotherapy for patients with many major mental disorders, such as schizophrenia, bipolar disorder, and major depression (American Psychiatric Association 2002, 2004, 2010). Many empirical studies indicate that patients who receive both psychopharmacolog-ical treatment and psychotherapy may have better treatment outcomes than patients who receive only psychopharmacological treatment for a number of conditions, including major depression (Hollon et al. 2014; Karyotaki et al. 2016), anxiety (Barlow et al. 2000; Fansi et al. 2015), bipolar disorder (Parikh et al. 2015), dependence/smoking cessation (Stead et al. 2016; U.S. Department of Health and Human Services 2000), and erectile dysfunction after radical prostatectomy (Naccarato et al. 2016). Preliminary evidence suggests that quality of life and functioning is improved with combined pharmacological and psychosocial treatments for depression (Kamenov et al. 2017), for borderline personality disorder (Bozzatello and Bellino 2016), and for some substance use disorders (Stead et al. 2016). The combination of pharmacotherapy and psychotherapy has thus been recommended in some guidelines, such as the National Institute for Health and Care Excellence guideline for the treatment and management of depression in adults.

To provide state-of-the-art clinical care for mental disorders, it is important that psychiatrists and psychiatric residents be able to provide the appropriate type of treatment or, more properly, the appropriate combination of treatments to address the patient's needs in accordance with known evidence related to the patient's diagnosis. Because an understanding of both pharmacological and psychotherapeutic approaches is such an important part of psychiatric practice, psychiatry residency training programs have given explicit attention to these topics for many years in their teaching and assessment of residents (Epstein and Hundert 2002). Rigorous psychiatric training should facilitate the mastery of skills for performing psychotherapy and administering psychopharmacology and should entail supervision on clinical cases. In practice, psychiatric trainees should become capable of providing both forms of treatment directly, as well as in a collaborative and/or in a supervisory capacity with other health care professionals. Combining psychopharmacology and psychotherapy is not a simple matter, however. Assessing patient needs, determining which professionals should provide the specific kind of treatment, and orchestrating the sequence and timing of the combination of treatments (i.e., which modality to start first or starting both at the same time) can be complicated and depends on the circumstances of the patient's mental health care. We begin with the most complex issue: how the patient initially presents for treatment and how the patient's presentation affects the provision of psychotherapy, psychopharmacology, neither, or both.

Psychiatric Triage: The System Has Become Confusing

Psychiatric triage has become very confusing for both patients and clinicians. Most patients are no longer able to call a psychiatrist or therapist directly and make an appointment for an evaluation. More often than not, patients are required to call an intake worker via their managed care or insurance provider, are asked to give historical and symptom information over the telephone, and then are directed to a clinical site for an evaluation. If the patient's symptoms are not acute, the patient may first be seen by a clinician or staff person who is not a physician but who will decide whether or not the patient should be seen by a physician for an evaluation, for medication, or for some other medical intervention. The decision regarding the need for medication might be made by the nonphysician at the initial evaluation or might be made sometime later. A physician psychiatrist who provides medications may be referred to as the *prescribing psychiatrist*.

When a patient is seen by a therapist and a physician is brought in to provide psychotropic medication and other consultation, the treatment is called "split treatment" or "collaborative treatment," depending on the level of coordination between the two clinicians. *Collaborative treatment* (Riba and Balon 1999) is the preferred term, because it describes what is ideal and preferable, but *split treatment* may often better capture the fragmentation that occurs in current systems of care. For these reasons, we denote this type of care as split/collaborative care to remind us of the problems inherent in having more than one provider and the need for communication.

If the patient sees a psychiatrist for the initial evaluation and remains with the psychiatrist for both psychotherapy and psychotropic medication, this is called *integrated treatment*. Similarly, if the patient is initially triaged to a therapist and is then referred to a psychiatrist who takes over both the psychotherapy and medication, this would also be integrated treatment.

Also, in many states, nurse practitioners and physician assistants are able to prescribe medications under the supervision of a physician. Therefore, a psychiatrist may be the supervising psychiatrist, but not the treating psychiatrist, for patients who are under the care of nurse practitioners and physician assistants. In addition, at the time of this writing, many states, including Iowa, Illinois, Louisiana, and New Mexico, and the U.S. Public Health Service, the U.S. military, and the territory of Guam have all given prescribing privileges to psychologists. In these contexts, psychologists must comply with the varying details of the scope of prescribing privileges and with the required curricular preparation and clinical training. Prescribing psychologists also must usually maintain a collaborative relationship with the patient's physician to comply with standards of care in most communities. The role of psychiatrists in providing supervision or oversight to psychologists with prescribing privileges is not consistent across these states and settings.

What is so confusing about these forms of split/collaborative versus integrated care? There are many issues to consider:

- Triage is often based on insurance or ability to pay rather than clinical needs or criteria.
- Access issues for mental health care make it difficult to provide the ideal match of patient, disorder, and symptoms with care provider. For example, a patient with treatment-resistant depression or bipolar disorder may not be able to see a specialist despite the severity of illness and may instead be matched to a general clinician.
- Many managed behavioral-care intermediaries are judged according to the number of days that elapse before patients are seen after their initial call for help or after discharge from the hospital. This system encourages patients to be seen by the first available clinician rather than by the best clinician for that particular patient.
- Insurance plans frequently impose limits on the total number of psychotherapy or psychopharmacology encounters in a certain time period, which may produce tensions and negotiations between the patient and treating specialist or between the psychiatrist and mental health worker (e.g., Would it be better to use these benefits for psychotherapy?). Some insurance companies complicate the process even more by not allowing patients to have a psychotherapy session and a medication review on the same day.
- Patients do not necessarily get the kind of treatment that they request or prefer in many systems of care and under many insurance entities. Patients may wish to see a psychiatrist, for example, but depending on the symptoms with which they are presenting, they may not see a psychiatrist, at least initially.
- Oftentimes, the initial triage for mental health services is done over the telephone by workers from a wide variety of backgrounds, not necessarily by licensed mental health practitioners.

Issues such as these complicate the conduct of high-quality clinical care for individuals in need of mental health services. Unfortunately, little research has been conducted on optimal approaches in access to care. We do know, however, that many individuals in need delay seeking care because of stigma, apprehension about navigating systems of care, and misunderstandings of the value of mental health services. The above-mentioned issues, such as nonstandardized procedures for initiating care, can contribute to these challenges for patients. Unfortunately, at this time, there is no platform to facilitate collaboration among the professions (e.g., psychiatry, psychology, social work, primary care) to evaluate the best ways to triage and manage the issues of integrated versus split/collaborative treatments. Such work would be immensely valuable, considering the prevalence of mental disorders and the dramatically increasing numbers of individuals seeking mental health services.

Many questions related to care seeking and split/collaborative care warrant empirical study. For example, the role of the primary care physician as gatekeeper for diagnosing and triaging patients for psychotherapy and pharmacotherapy continues to be a major and important area of study. It continues to be difficult for primary care physicians to sort out psychiatric symptoms in the short amount of face-to-face time they have with patients. The physical symptoms with which patients often present (e.g., back pain, headache, fatigue) are difficult to distinguish from depressive and anxiety symptoms. Furthermore, it is often a challenge for primary care physicians to arrange for patients to be seen by qualified mental health professionals in a timely fashion. In addition, the field of psychiatry is undergoing increased specialization with the emergence of the formally recognized subspecialties of geriatric psychiatry, child and adolescent psychiatry, substance use/addiction medicine, forensic psychiatry, and consultation-liaison psychiatry (formerly psychosomatic medicine). Subspecialty care needs of patients may contribute to the complexity faced by primary care clinicians who are deciding whether to provide care directly or to incorporate integrated or split/collaborative treatment approaches. Furthermore, evidence-informed guidelines for making the choice are still lacking. A third category of issues that merits empirical study relates to the inclusion of telehealth or digital health components of care. For example, in some circumstances (e.g., rural communities), psychiatric care may not be available except through remote consultation or telepsychiatry services. To our knowledge, the impact of this situation has not been properly studied.

The issues listed above are complex and not easily resolved. As a first step, however, we wish to highlight that every psychiatrist and psychiatric resident should learn about the triage system that is in place in each clinical care site where he or she works. Moreover, for clinical training, we suggest the following as a competency:

Competency

Psychiatry residents should demonstrate an appreciation for the triage system that is in place at their institution for both inpatient and outpatient psychotherapy and psychopharmacological treatments.

As illustrated in this chapter, even the initial triage system that begins the entry or route to care for the patient is complex and may introduce considerable burdens for the patient who is already dealing with the burden of illness and distress. For convenience or logistics, the patient might want to see just one clinician for both medication and psychotherapy, but because of the nature of the system, the patient might end up seeing two clinicians. Interestingly, because this arrangement may or may not be less expensive than seeing one clinician (Dewan 1999; Goldman et al. 1998), health care costs might not be the primary driving agent for this type of care.

During split/collaborative care, the therapist and the physician might have a history of working with each other, or they might not. The system of care might be closed, meaning that the clinicians in the system know each other and work with one another. Examples of closed systems are a university outpatient psychiatry clinic and a community mental health clinic. Alternatively, the system might be open, and the clinicians might not regularly collaborate with one another. Factors might include geography: if a patient is in an area where there is an abundance of therapists but very few psychiatrists or primary care clinicians, the patient may have to travel a long distance to receive care from a physician. In such a case, there may be less of a chance that the therapist and physician have worked together. Similarly, in an area with a large population of both therapists and physicians, there may also be less of a chance that the clinicians have worked together.

Added to these factors are many others that make the triage—and therefore the decision about split/collaborative versus integrated care—very confusing and complex. Is the patient a child, an adolescent, or an older adult? Does the patient have a co-occurring medical condition that would affect whether it would be best for him or her to receive both psychotherapy and medication in an integrated care model? Does the patient have a substance use problem? Are there psychosocial factors, family issues, a history of nonadherence to treatment, or belief systems regarding psychotherapy or medication that might have an impact on whether split/collaborative treatment or integrated treatment would be best for the patient? What personal or other factors would be important for the clinician to understand in the triage process?

Competency

Psychiatry residents should be able to demonstrate the ability to take a history regarding factors that would influence the decision to provide the patient with split/collaborative versus integrated treatment.

Thinking About Integrated Treatment Versus Split/Collaborative Treatment

The pathway for a patient in need of services to obtain evaluation by a clinician is no longer straightforward and is very dependent on a host of factors, many of which are not clinically important but are more dependent on fiscal, geographic, and insurance considerations. It is therefore incumbent on the practicing psychiatrist or psychiatry resident to take heed of these factors in trying to understand and then assess what is best for the patient regarding integrated versus split/collaborative treatment.

Given that there are currently no standards or guidelines for determining these issues for patients based on age, diagnostic categories, and comorbidities, how should the resident begin to differentiate and think about choosing between integrated and split/collaborative treatment for a specific patient? This question is especially germane, because it is unlikely that the resident is conducting the initial telephone (or telepsychiatry) evaluation or triage; he or she may instead be picking up the patient's case at some point after psychotherapy has already been started by another therapist.

Because this confusing system of triage and evaluation has arguably become the norm in today's current psychiatric practice—in managed care settings, community mental health settings, and even in university ambulatory care settings—it is very important that the psychiatrist or psychiatry resident be armed with the tools to understand the issues. Furthermore, beyond understanding, it is necessary to provide ways to determine competency regarding both split/collaborative treatment and integrated treatment on the part of the general psychiatry resident by the time of graduation.

The Residency Review Committee of the Accreditation Council for Graduate Medical Education (American Medical Association 2004) has published requirements regarding competencies in five areas of psychotherapy. The general resident should demonstrate competency in all these areas of psychotherapy by the time of graduation. Each residency program has had to develop a method of testing and evaluating residents on their ability and mastery of these requirements. Initially, one required competency was psychotherapy combined with psychopharmacology. The Residency Review Committee was nondirective as to whether psychotherapy and psychopharmacology should be provided in the integrated treatment model or in the split/collaborative treatment model. Unfortunately, in later revisions of the Program Requirements for Psychiatry, the Residency Review Committee removed specific requirements for two psychotherapy modalities, one of them being psychotherapy combined with pharmacotherapy. The rationale for the removal is not clear. It is possible that the committee believed that the combination of pharmacotherapy and psychotherapy should be a commonly required skill and did not feel that it should be codified in any specific way. Nevertheless, the current Program Requirements for Psychiatry state that residents must demonstrate competence in "managing and treating patients using pharmacological regimes, including concurrent use of medications and psychotherapy."

In this book, therefore, one of our goals is to provide guidance for assessing the competency of residents to provide both split/collaborative treatment and integrated treatment. We believe it is important that psychiatry residents understand the principles, issues, factors, and dynamics that affect patients who enter the psychiatric system for evaluation and that influence whether patients remain in split/collaborative treatment or integrated treatment.

As an example, a patient may change jobs while undergoing split/collaborative treatment with a therapist and a psychiatrist. The new employer's insurance provider could dictate that the patient change providers and be seen by just one clinician. The patient might then decide to be seen by just the psychiatrist for integrated treatment. The psychiatrist must be able to adjust care accordingly and discuss the new situation (including insurance/financial arrangements) with the patient. Similarly, a patient might be in split/collaborative treatment and not be doing well clinically, experiencing serious symptoms and being impaired in his or her employment situation. The psychiatrist must be able to determine the causes for this situation and determine if the patient would be better managed with integrated treatment. The psychiatrist, therefore, should be able to manage patients, understand factors, and easily move between integrated and split/collaborative treatment. Throughout residency, competencies for both integrated and split/collaborative treatment ideally would be taught to all psychiatry residents, and all psychiatry residents would be evaluated by the time of graduation.

In this book, we mainly focus on competencies in adult psychiatry in the outpatient setting. We recognize that inpatient units also provide split/collaborative treatment. Certain patient populations (e.g., children, older patients) require split/collaborative treatment in a different, unique format because parents, other medical professionals, and caregivers are involved and because different types of consent and cognitive issues are germane, among other reasons. There are also certain diagnostic categories (e.g., substance abuse, psychosomatic medicine, forensics) that lend themselves to different types of split/collaborative treatment, which calls for unique competencies. The scope of this book is limited primarily to adult outpatient psychiatry competencies.

Stages of Psychiatry Residency: Historical Perspective and Current Generalities Regarding Training Patterns

Psychiatry training, as Brenner (2016) notes, should yield "doctors who are prepared to guide the treatment team in attention to the whole patient through the integration of diverse treatment modalities" (p. 745). The 4-year curriculum of psychiatry residency provides a platform for the growth in knowledge and skills of early career physician specialists so that they are able to provide clinical care competently and compassionately.

Years 1 and 2

Psychiatry residency training is developmental: residents gradually receive more independence in their learning and supervision. Much of the first 2 years of the 4-year course of study have traditionally been hospital based, involving some of the most seriously ill patients but with more intensive, on-site supervision. During the first year of residency, 6 months of study in medicine and neurology are required. Eight (6–16) months of training are required on general psychiatric wards and child and adolescent, geriatric, addiction, consultation/liaison psychiatry, and psychiatric emergency services rotations along with other required experiences. Because the first 2 years of training are often focused on acutely ill hospitalized patients, there is not much time for longitudinal combined psychotherapy and pharmacotherapy experience.

Although some residency programs have tried to incorporate more outpatient and longitudinal rotations into the first 2 years—frequently in the form of a continuity clinic a few hours a week—it is often difficult to do so because of factors such as resident work-hour rules, the imperative to conform to license requirements, financial reimbursement for residents' time based on providing care on inpatient hospital services, and the need to supervise residents more closely using hospital attending psychiatrists.

Because psychiatry residents spend most of their first 2 years on inpatient units (either psychiatric, primary care, or neurological), on a practical basis, residents are very engaged in split/collaborative treatment. The inpatient psychiatric ward, for example, is an excellent representation of the collaborative work of nurses, who provide much of the direct medical and sometimes psychotherapeutic management; social workers, who provide psychotherapy as well as discharge planning; primary care physicians, general internists, and specialists, who deliver much of the care related to physical medicine; psychologists, who provide psychotherapy as well as psychological testing; psychiatrists, who serve as attending psychiatrists; and residents, who are junior to the psychiatrists. The psychiatrists provide medication management; other medical services such as electroconvulsive treatment; and overall leadership, evaluation, diagnosis, discharge, and so on.

This team-based collaborative model has been historically quite pervasive since the onset of general hospital psychiatry. Up until the last 25 years, however, much of the psychotherapy in the general hospital had been provided by the psychiatry resident or attending psychiatrist. At this point in time, the length of stay of hospitalized patients has decreased dramatically for both physically ill and mentally ill individuals, and the criteria for admitting patients to the hospital have become much more narrow (i.e., acute suicidality, acute psychosis, and acute agitation). In short, the inpatient psychiatry model remains very much a split/collaborative model, but the resident and attending psychiatrist are providing much less of the psychotherapy to the inpatients than in previous years. The length of stay on the inpatient psychiatric unit has become so brief that by necessity the psychiatry resident and attending psychiatrist have become less able to provide face-to-face psychotherapy, and, instead, they provide more of the medication or other medical management.

The nature of the inpatient psychiatry unit has changed dramatically and so has the role of the psychiatry resident. Residents must be able to provide both integrated and split/collaborative treatment to patients who have major and acute psychiatric problems. They must be able to work collaboratively with a number of professionals in providing patients with care and must make determinations for patients to be discharged into settings that will provide outpatient psychiatric care. The psychiatry resident and attending psychiatrist must determine—based on a range of fiscal, geographic, and other factors—whether the patient should be discharged into integrated treatment or into split/collaborative treatment. With most of the first 2 years of residency taking place in the inpatient setting or the psychiatric emergency service, how can the resident learn to make such decisions for outpatient care? What are the guiding principles for making these determinations? What are the dependent and independent factors that should be addressed and documented in the decision-making process?

It is important for residents to learn the skills of triage in years 1 and 2, when they are working in psychiatric emergency departments and on inpatient units and are making plans for patients to be seen as outpatients. Residents should achieve competence in triaging patients for either integrated or split/collaborative treatment or care within their second or third year of training, when residents are providing more outpatient care.

Years 3 and 4

In many psychiatry programs, the third year of residency training provides the bulk of the continuous outpatient year. Residents are usually assigned to an outpatient clinic for most of the time but also may have to meet requirements in specialty areas—for example, geriatric, child and adolescent, and community mental health—if they did not meet them in previous years or if they decide to make their fourth year part of their child and adolescent residency training. Residents are often very busy during this year with scheduling of patients, clinics, supervision, and core didactics. In addition, more and more residents are thinking about subspecialty training in child and adolescent psychiatry, so during the third year these residents are interviewing for child and adolescent psychiatry training programs that start in their fourth year of residency. Some residents also become more involved in scholarly activities and research to be competitive when applying for various fellowships and jobs. This broad set of duties and activities makes it very important for the resident and the residency training director to ensure that all year-appropriate requirements and competencies are met by the end of the third year of residency training.

It is during the third year of residency training that the issues of split/collaborative treatment versus integrated treatment are highlighted. In many residency programs, third-year residents begin the year with a list of patients—handed down by the previous residents—for whom medication, not psychotherapy, needs to be provided. The lists of such patients are often long, many of the patients have not been seen for months, and the diagnoses of these patients have remained the same for years.

In some clinics, an attending psychiatrist will not have seen these medication-management patients for years. The medication-management patients may or may not be seen by therapists for psychotherapy, and their therapists may or may not be within the university system. If the patient is receiving psychotherapy from a therapist within the university system and the resident is seeing the patient for medication management, this would be considered split/collaborative treatment. If the patient is being seen by a therapist outside the university system, it is still a split/collaborative treatment arrangement, but collaboration and communication are much more difficult. If the patient is seen by the resident only for medication, this might be called integrated treatment, although some residents might not view providing psychotherapy as part of their role.

During the third year of training, residents see, and engage in integrated and split/collaborative treatment in various settings involving, patients with a wide range of ages and diagnoses (e.g., children, older adults, patients in community mental health settings). Supervision is also quite variable. Faculty members tend to supervise residents—and the residents' cases—while managing large caseloads. This is often difficult to do.

Supervision of long-term psychodynamic psychotherapy, often conducted in private practitioners' offices, focuses on dynamic issues, not historically on medication or split/collaborative treatment cases. In the community mental health system, residents rely greatly on case workers and social workers for information on patients' social, occupational, and family supports. The child psychiatry setting is very much based on a collaborative model, relying on input from social workers, psychologists, and school staff. The same may be said for the geriatric setting, where there is a medical model of collaborative care. The Veterans Health Administration, with its emphasis on large-team collaboration and not-so-flexible bureaucracy, also poses its own challenges for residents.

Third-year competencies are strongly related to the various types of patients, settings, and systems in which the resident is working. Core lectures often do not focus on issues of integrated versus split/collaborative treatment, but instead focus on psychopharmacology directly or psychotherapy history and techniques.

How residents decide which patients to keep and which to give up as they progress through their training is a critical matter to be determined with an overall supervisor. The problem is that in many residency programs, there may not be an overall supervisor who knows about all the residents' cases, which makes this holistic review more difficult. Unfortunately, supervision throughout the third year in many residency programs can be quite fragmented. Logs or casebooks are frequently not detailed enough to reflect the complexity of combined psychotherapy and pharmacotherapy. The upper limits of the numbers of split/ collaborative treatment cases or integrated treatment cases a resident should carry during the third year or fourth year or by the time of graduation have not yet been determined for the discipline of psychiatry.

Some university clinics, for example, recommend that third-year residents try to refer stable patients back to their primary care physicians for medication management at the end of the year. There are many reasons for this recommendation: 1) too many patients will be on the list for the incoming third-year residents; 2) in a capitated system it is not economical to see patients more frequently, so the university psychiatry clinic loses money every time residents see such patients; and 3) depending on the insurance carrier, there might not be any reimbursement for residents' time when they see medication-management patients (this depends on whether there is an attending supervisor who is also seeing the patient). Interestingly, the question of whether these economic issues should be factors in making decisions about educational issues has not been properly addressed by the discipline of psychiatry. Should a resident necessarily be reimbursed for services when his or her salary is supposedly paid from other sources? Complex issues such as these provide further evidence of the need to carefully evaluate the competency of residents as they complete this very intensive year of providing split/collaborative treatment and integrated treatment in various settings.

The fourth year of training is relatively flexible and may be a good time for residents to review and consolidate skills in integrated versus split/collaborative treatment. By then, residents have had a good overview of both inpatient and outpatient split/collaborative and integrated treatment in various settings with patients of all ages and comorbidities. A potential problem with this fourth year of residency training, however, is its heterogeneity. The flexibility of this year makes the experience different from one resident to another and from one program to another. Often residents use the fourth year for taking electives, doing research, or sharpening their skills in a particular area. Also, if the resident chooses to enter child and adolescent psychiatry, the fourth year is commonly spent in training for this subspecialty. Thus, the fourth year is somewhat inconsistent, and residents often choose rotations that might enable them to enter advanced training in forensics, geriatrics, or other areas. Moreover, some programs require that residents keep several psychotherapy cases during year 4; however, these cases are probably mostly integrated ones, with residents providing both psychotherapy and pharmacotherapy. The split/collaborative treatment experience during year 4 may be very limited.

The fourth year has not traditionally been a time when residents are thinking of honing their skills in integrated versus split/collaborative treatment. Residents are thinking instead about jobs and the transition to practice. Many of the higher-paying jobs require clinicians to see many patients for evaluations for medication in a short period of time. Such jobs are in systems of care or clinics where the triage for the evaluation comes from a social worker or psychologist within the system. In these positions, the psychiatrist must do a lot of medication evaluations and patient follow-up in a split/collaborative treatment arrangement. Using an integrated model for patient follow-up is usually not the preferred arrangement in many cost-sensitive health care systems.

Residents in their fourth year are often confronted with choices about whether or not to take such jobs. Residents are generally carrying large debts from their medical school loans, so high-paying, salaried jobs for this kind of split/collaborative treatment work are certainly tantalizing. Whether or not residents interested in these jobs go back and ask for more split/collaborative treatment cases within their residency programs has not been well studied. The positions being offered to residents on graduation—whether they are in clinics, closed systems of care, or community mental health centers—often require more skills in split/collaborative treatment. Ensuring that residents are prepared to safely take on such positions is clearly one of the reasons why improved assessment of competencies and skills is needed.

Summary

Psychiatric practice involves the ability to provide care for patients within the context of integrated and split/collaborative care models. Patients face many burdens and complexities as they seek care for mental health needs. Psychiatrists and psychiatric residents may be brought into patient care early or not; the process of referring patients for care with a psychiatrist is inconsistent.

The success of residents in learning how to deliver treatment in the context of integrated and split/collaborative models relates to the curricular experiences and the professional developmental sequence of the residency; the type and quality of supervision provided; the core lecture and other didactic experiences; and the clinical experiences and settings and the numbers of patients with certain types of diagnoses, ages, comorbidities, and so on. How do all of these clinical and didactic experiences get integrated so that the resident can see the differences and similarities between split/collaborative and integrated treatment? Given the historical changes that have affected inpatient and outpatient care practices and subspecialty training in the last 25 years, have general adult residency training programs kept up with the ability to evaluate skills and competencies in integrated versus split/collaborative treatment? Are residents in both adult and child psychiatry training programs being adequately prepared for their future jobs?

This book is meant to help with the assessment of competencies of psychiatrists and psychiatric residents in the practice of integrated and split/collaborative care, a type of assessment that was introduced several years ago and yet does not have a substantial evidence base. We hope that the ideas set forth in these pages will serve to move those in the field to discuss, study, and improve the methods of training psychiatrists and psychiatric residents and of assessing their skills and competencies so that they will be better prepared to provide excellent psychotherapeutic and pharmacotherapeutic care, whether in split/ collaborative or integrated treatment.

References

American Medical Association: ACGME program requirements for residency-education in psychiatry, in Graduate Medical Education Directory, 2004–2005. Chicago, IL, American Medical Association, 2004, pp 369–370

American Psychiatric Association: Practice Guideline for the Treatment of Patients With Bipolar Disorder, 2nd Edition. Washington, DC, American Psychiatric Publishing, 2002

American Psychiatric Association: Practice Guideline for the Treatment of Patients With Schizophrenia, 2nd Edition. Washington, DC, American Psychiatric Publishing, 2004

American Psychiatric Association: American Psychiatric Association Practice Guideline for the Treatment of Patients With Major Depressive Disorder, 3rd Edition. Washington, DC, American Psychiatric Publishing, 2010

Barlow DH, Gorman JM, Shear MK, et al: Cognitive-behavioral therapy, imipramine, or their combination for panic disorder: a randomized controlled trial. JAMA 283(19):2529–2536, 2000 10815116

Bozzatello P, Bellino S: Combined therapy with interpersonal psychotherapy adapted for borderline personality disorder: a two-years follow-up. Psychiatry Res 240:151–156, 2016 27107668

Brenner AM: Revisiting the biopsychosocial formulation: neuroscience, social science, and the patient's subjective experience. Acad Psychiatry 40(5):740–746, 2016 27060094

Correll CU, Kratochvil CJ, March JS: Developments in pediatric psychopharmacology: focus on stimulants, antidepressants, and antipsychotics. J Clin Psychiatry 72(5):655–670, 20111 21658348

Dewan M: Are psychiatrists cost-effective? An analysis of integrated versus split treatment. Am J Psychiatry 156(2):324–326, 1999 9989575

Epstein RM, Hundert EM: Defining and assessing professional competence. JAMA 287(2):226–235, 2002 11779266

Fansi A, Jehanno C, Lapalme M, et al: Effectiveness of psychotherapy compared to pharmacotherapy for the treatment of anxiety and depressive disorders in adults: A literature review [in French]. Sante Ment Que 40(4):141–173, 2015 27203537

Goldman W, McCulloch J, Cuffel B, et al: Outpatient utilization patterns of integrated and split psychotherapy and pharmacotherapy for depression. Psychiatr Serv 49(4):477–482, 1998 9550237

Hollon SD, DeRubeis RJ, Fawcett J, et al: Effect of cognitive therapy with antidepressant medications vs antidepressants alone on the rate of recovery in major depressive disorder: a randomized clinical trial. JAMA Psychiatry 71(10):1157–1164, 2014 25142196

Kamenov K, Twomey C, Cabello M, et al: The efficacy of psychotherapy, pharmacotherapy and their combination on functioning and quality of life in depression: a meta-analysis. Psychol Med 47(3):414–425, 2017 27780478

Karyotaki E, Smit Y, Holdt Henningsen K, et al: Combining pharmacotherapy and psychotherapy or monotherapy for major depression? A meta-analysis on the long-term effects. J Affect Disord 194:144–152, 2016 26826534

Katon WJ, Unützer J: Health reform and the Affordable Care Act: the importance of mental health treatment to achieving the triple aim. J Psychosom Res 74(6):533–537, 2013 23731753

Naccarato AM, Reis LO, Ferreira U, et al: Psychotherapy and phosphodiesterase-5 inhibitor in early rehabilitation after radical prostatectomy: a prospective randomised controlled trial. Andrologia 48(10):1183–1187, 2016 27062069

Olfson M, Blanco C, Liu SM, et al: National trends in the office-based treatment of children, adolescents, and adults with antipsychotics. Arch Gen Psychiatry 69(12):1247–1256, 2012 22868273

Olfson M, Blanco C, Wang S, et al: National trends in the mental health care of children, adolescents, and adults by office-based physicians. JAMA Psychiatry 71(1):81–90, 2014 24285382

Parikh SV, Hawke LD, Velyvis V, et al: Combined treatment: impact of optimal psychotherapy and medication in bipolar disorder. Bipolar Disord 17(1):86–96, 2015 25046246

Raney LE: Integrating primary care and behavioral health: The role of the psychiatrist in the collaborative care model. Am J Psychiatry 172(8):721–728, 2015 26234599

Riba MB, Balon R (eds): Psychopharmacology and Psychotherapy: A Collaborative Approach. Washington, DC, American Psychiatric Press, 1999

Stead LF, Koilpillai P, Fanshawe TR, et al: Combined pharmacotherapy and behavioural interventions for smoking cessation. Cochrane Database Syst Rev 3:CD008286, 2016 27009521

U.S. Department of Health and Human Services: Reducing Tobacco Use: A Report of the Surgeon General. Atlanta, GA, Centers for Disease Control and Prevention, 2000

Selection of Medication and Psychotherapy in Integrated Treatment

2

Thinking About the Issues in Integrated Treatment

Some of the difficulties regarding integrated versus split/collaborative treatment relate to the following issues: 1) how patients are triaged; 2) who does the initial evaluation and makes the diagnosis (e.g., a referring clinician or resident/attending physician); 3) the experience of the clinician in various types of psychotherapy; 4) the goals, commitment, and resources of the patient; 5) the level of patient understanding of various treatments (either preconceived knowledge achieved through various means or understanding achieved through discussion and psychoeducation during the initial session); and 6) what the clinician(s) can reasonably hope to accomplish. Whether the patient is recommended for integrated treatment or split/collaborative treatment, questions about the type of psychotherapy and medication usage (whether or not to use medication, when to administer it, what type to use) are clearly relevant factors. In this chapter, we discuss the provision of medication and psychotherapy in an integrated model: the psychiatry resident is providing both the psychotherapy and the medication management or other medical care.

When the Patients Calls
for an Appointment

A patient calls for an appointment when he or she is having a problem. The patient may have some expectations about what he or she might need based on personal history, the experiences of friends or family members with similar (or different) problems, portrayals in the media, or a clinician recommendation. Or perhaps the patient has no expectations and simply wants help.

As described by Bender and Messner (2003, p. 9), the initial call may be challenging both for the novice therapist and for the patient. The patient's privacy and concerns should be kept in mind (Bender and Messner 2003, p. 9). The initial call is usually focused on scheduling the initial session and determining whether insurance will cover costs, unless this was already done by the office or billing clerk. A realistic time frame for the initial session should be provided— the time should be suitable for both the patient and the resident without the necessity of rushing in and out—and the length and cost of the session should also be specified.

The doctor–patient relationship begins with the telephone call for the initial appointment, and whoever speaks with the patient to schedule the appointment acts as an extension of the physician (Simon 2004). It is important for that person to ask the patient about what led to making the call for the appointment and, as part of the history taking, what beliefs and issues the patient has that will need to be sorted out with the psychiatry resident.

The first moments of the session are very important, although they certainly may be anxiety provoking for the patient and for the resident or attending physician. The patient may analyze the way he or she is greeted; thus, addressing the patient in the waiting area should be done in a way to preserve the patient's confidentiality. The patient may also analyze how the resident looks (the resident's facial expression and dress), whether or not the resident shakes the patient's hand, and how the waiting room and office are decorated (e.g., whether there are any personal items in the office). First impressions count in almost every situation, and this is certainly true in the interaction between the doctor and the patient.

Patients often come in with biases, and it is helpful to understand these along with the patients' belief systems (Carli 1999) regarding medication and psychotherapy. For example, some have had successes with psychotropic medication or other types of medication (e.g., antibiotics) in the past and therefore might be more open to thinking about medication. If patients have had adverse medication reactions, allergic reactions, or serious side effects from medications, discussing these issues will be important.

Patients may be quite frightened about their symptoms and what they imagine or fear about seeing a psychiatrist. There are many stigmatizing portrayals in movies, television, and other media in which seeing a psychiatrist is represented as a scary event with frightening consequences such as being locked up, being placed in a straitjacket, being immediately administered electroconvulsive therapy, or being put in a diabetic coma. Although most patients probably will not be worried about such things, it certainly will behoove the resident to assess these issues and begin to allay the patient's fears and worries.

Questions to consider asking the patient include the following:

1. Why did you decide to see someone?
2. When did you decide to call for an appointment?
3. With whom did you speak to arrange the appointment?
4. Did you encounter any difficulties in making or getting this appointment?
5. What was your overall experience with the call?
6. Do you have any ideas about what might happen here? What do you expect to achieve here?

These are open-ended questions that might help elicit issues, thoughts, and feelings that will be important to understand. If these questions are not asked early on, it is sometimes difficult to go back and retrieve the important information.

Competency

Psychiatry residents should be able to demonstrate the ability to ask questions regarding why the patient is being seen for a psychiatric evaluation (potentially for medication and psychotherapy).

Thinking Broadly

The initial evaluation between the resident and the patient is discussed in Chapter 3, "Evaluation and Opening in Integrated Treatment." What we focus on here is that too often the resident is worried about trying to make the diagnosis in the first session with the patient. It could be that the patient has already received a diagnosis from another clinician. Certainly, after seeing the patient, the resident ideally should do a dictation and arrive at a diagnosis (not only for billing purposes but also to formulate a management plan to review with the supervisor).

But from the patient's point of view, the objective of the first session is often to establish comfort with and trust in the resident. The patient wants to know if the resident has the ability, empathy, skill, and experience to be able to help the patient with his or her symptoms. Does this resident understand what has brought the patient to the clinic? Does the resident seem interested in the patient? And if there is some feeling that the resident does understand, what is the hook or draw that will bring the patient back to be seen for follow-up?

The first session between the patient and the resident is critically important because the resident must demonstrate his or her ability to care for the patient. The patient may or may not have expectations of what the resident is supposed to do or what the resident will be doing. The resident should have the skills not only to grasp what is going on in the room during the initial session but also to impart a sense of confidence without overwhelming the patient. The resident ideally should provide a focus for future sessions and give the patient a reason why he or she should return. This is a lot of work and takes a lot of skill.

The questions that the patient asks during the initial session may be about psychotherapy: Will a couch be used? Will the patient be hypnotized or hospitalized? Will the patient's spouse be asked to join in the sessions? How much will the patient be asked to reveal? How often will the patient need to come to sessions, and for how long—months or years? What is the resident's availability, and will the patient even be seeing the resident for follow-up? What is the goal of therapy? Does therapy usually help? The patient may also ask questions about medication: Will the patient be forced to take medication? Will it be something like what the patient's sibling or friend has taken? What will medication help with (e.g., mood, anxiety, sleep, fatigue)? What are the side effects? Will the medication have an impact on sexuality? How long will the patient need to take the medication? How much will it cost?

Often, especially during training years 1–3, the resident may be nervous about the evaluation as well. It is very difficult to make an assessment or diagnosis, decide on some sort of treatment plan, form an alliance with the patient, and feel that there are enough "hooks" that the patient will return for a follow-up appointment. Added to these tasks are decisions that the resident must make regarding the type of psychotherapy (e.g., cognitive-behavioral therapy, interpersonal therapy, psychodynamic therapy) that may benefit the patient, the skill level that the resident possesses to perform the needed psychotherapy, and whether or not medication needs to be discussed and prescribed at the initial interview.

During the initial interview, the resident is engaged in psychotherapy: beginning the doctor–patient relationship; forming an alliance with the patient; learning to understand the resources, coping mechanisms, strengths, and weaknesses of the patient; and setting an agenda for future sessions. Whether the focus of the session is on medication, diagnosis, or other issues, the resident should show competence, confidence, and ability to gauge the patient's capacity for self-reflection and goal setting and should determine whether or not the patient is ready to take the next steps. The patient's safety must also always be assessed and evaluated. Although the first session should start with open-ended questions, the time restriction will require that the resident become more directive. Note writing should not be extensive and should be explained to the patient in a positive fashion.

These are very difficult concepts for the resident to master. If the resident wishes to talk about medication, a diagnosis needs to be made beforehand. For example, the resident cannot talk about prescribing an antidepressant medication without talking with the patient about a mood disorder. So, the resident needs to determine whether the patient is ready to listen to and accept this type of discussion. Similarly, if there is a mood disorder and interpersonal psychotherapy would also be part of the treatment, the resident needs to decide whether to discuss what this type of psychotherapy entails, how many visits are required, the goals of treatment, and how the psychotherapy relates to taking medication. The resident also needs to find a way to gauge the patient's capacity for change (Beitman et al. 2003).

As noted by Bush and Sandberg (2012), one needs to consider many additional questions regarding the need and relative efficacy of combined treatment. Some of these questions may be applied to the immediate clinical situation of the first session. What types of patients may require a combination approach and what types of patients may need only a single approach? What may be the value of sequencing the treatment versus starting both at the same time? Do some forms or subtypes of the illness benefit more from combined treatment than others (e.g., major depressive disorder vs. persistent depressive disorder)? What factors may moderate response to combined treatment?

The moderating factors also need to be assessed and factored into the treatment plan. For instance, there are two potential major moderators—personality disorders and trauma—that need to be addressed in order to answer the question of whether psychotherapy may be necessary in addition to medication (Bush and Sandberg 2012). Many clinicians have observed that depression accompanied by personality disorders is less responsive to treatment (Bush and Sandberg 2012). It is important to note that without a good history, it is almost impossible to diagnose a personality disorder. Patients with severe personality disorders not only may be less responsive to trauma, but these patients may also trigger various countertransference issues in their therapist and physician, which may further complicate their treatment. For instance, in a study by Colli et al. (2014), paranoid and antisocial personality disorders were associated with criticized/mistreated countertransference, and borderline personality disorder was related to helpless/inadequate, overwhelmed/disorganized, and special/overinvolved countertransference. In addition, disengaged countertransference was associated with schizotypal and narcissistic personality disorders and was negatively associated with dependent and histrionic personality disorders. Colli et al. (2014) also noted stronger negative feelings when working with lower-functioning patients.

In regard to trauma, Nemeroff and colleagues (2003), in their additional analysis of data from a study by Keller and colleagues (2000), observed that among chronically depressed patients, psychotherapy alone was superior to antidepressant monotherapy for individuals with a history of early childhood trauma (e.g., early loss of a parent, physical or sexual abuse, neglect). Moreover, the combination of psychotherapy and pharmacotherapy was only marginally superior to psychotherapy among the cohort of individuals with a history of childhood abuse. Nemeroff et al. (2003) noted that psychotherapy may be an essential element in the treatment of patients with chronic forms of major depression and a history of childhood trauma.

To summarize, the key ingredients in this first session regarding combined psychotherapy and medication include the following:

1. Forging a doctor–patient alliance
2. Inquiring about how the patient got to the first session
3. Asking about and listening to the patient's belief systems about medication and psychotherapy
4. Assessing the patient's capacity for discussion of the diagnosis, treatment plan, and types of therapy
5. Assessing the resident's own capacity to deliver the recommended type of treatment
6. Reassuring the patient about the confidential nature of the treatment, but also discussing situations in which confidentiality might be broken (e.g., posing a danger to oneself, posing a danger to others)
7. Inquiring about the patient's desired/imagined goals for treatment, medication, and psychotherapy
8. Engaging the patient in psychoeducation, when appropriate and necessary

As Donkers et al. (2009) noted, brief psychoeducation for depression and psychological distress can reduce symptoms, is easily implemented, can be immediately applied, and is not expensive. Psychoeducation may be the first intervention for those experiencing psychological distress.

Last but not least, as Bush and Sandberg (2012) recommended, when considering combined treatment for depression, the clinician should consider costs of treatments, patient preferences, clinical features of the illness, and complicating/moderating factors before recommending combined/integrated treatment, despite its edge in efficacy.

Medication: General Issues to Be Addressed

If medication is one of the treatments that may be of benefit to the patient, the resident should determine and address the following:

1. Is the patient motivated to use medication? If not, what factors are preventing the patient from considering medication (e.g., denial, externalization) (Tasman et al. 2000, p. 93)?
2. What are the target symptoms for the medication? Which symptoms are most distressing or important to the patient?

3. What are the comorbid medical or other diagnoses that might interact with or relate to the use of psychotropic medication (e.g., personality disorders [Bush and Sandberg 2012; Colli et al. 2014], psychological trauma [Nemeroff et al. 2003], chronic physical illnesses such as diabetes, or severe physical illnesses such as cancer)?
4. Which side effects of the medication might be most distressing to the patient or to the patient's family members?
5. What obstacles might impede taking the medication? Examples are scheduling of doses; the need for blood assays and laboratory visits; general problems with adherence to taking daily medication; difficulty swallowing; difficulty remembering to take medication; costs of medication; problems with work- or school-related functions (e.g., driving); and partner/family objection to or discouragement of taking medication.
6. What beliefs does the patient have about the medication? Does the patient believe that psychotropic medication is addictive or causes brain damage?

The resident needs to provide a fair amount of psychoeducation to the patient (and possibly to family members) when medication is prescribed. In some states, consent forms for administering medications must be signed by patients, and fact sheets about the medication and side effects must be provided and noted in the chart. These matters all take time, and the resident must gauge how much time there is in the session and how much time to use for all of these issues.

Patients and families cannot be hurried. As an example, it might be wise for the resident to begin the discussion of medication but to delay the actual prescribing of medication until the next visit, especially when the resident is not sure about the diagnosis. Information on the medication could be sent home with the patient, as well as information on the diagnosis (e.g., depression). Some patients might also benefit from being informed of good Web sites where additional information might be gleaned. Residents might want to be prepared to direct patients to such Internet sites (Hsiung 2002).

We find it increasingly useful to introduce the atmosphere of "shared decision." In this situation, the resident/physician discusses various medication options along with their pros and cons and explores the patient's preferences, beliefs, experiences, and biases, and then together they arrive at the most acceptable medication to be prescribed.

Factors That Affect the Prescribing of Medication

Residents need to assess their working alliance with each patient to make the use of medications and psychotherapy successful. In addition, there are other skill sets that are important for the prescribing of medication. For residents, the setting—inpatient versus outpatient—is an important factor.

Inpatient

In the inpatient setting, starting medications is easier for several reasons: the patient can be watched continuously for side effects, the medication is provided by a nurse on a regular schedule, and the cost of the medication is factored into the hospital stay. Often, there are groups for discussing medications; many patients are taking medication, so individual patients do not feel singled out; and because patients are not in their usual environment (e.g., home, the workplace), certain issues, such as the need to drive or to have quick reflexes, do not arise. There are also attending psychiatrists, nurses, and other professionals who can speak with the patient and with the family to reinforce the diagnosis and the need for medication with certain types of disorders. Studies have shown that the addition of psychotherapy (e.g., cognitive-behavioral therapy in the case of depressive disorders [Köhler et al. 2013]) may improve outcome over standard procedure in acute psychiatric treatment.

Residents are also very well supervised on inpatient units. The attending physician often makes suggestions as to the class, type, and dosage of medication to be used. Inpatient units often tend to use certain types of medication for sleep, anxiety, new-onset psychosis, depression, and so forth. There are certain prescribing patterns based on hospital formularies and what the attending physicians feel most comfortable with, based on their experiences and the types of patients usually treated in that setting. Residents tend to learn these basic medications, become comfortable prescribing them, and then build on this knowledge base.

On inpatient units, sleep patterns are monitored, appetite changes are evaluated by daily weighing and by noting food remaining on trays, and gastrointestinal side effects are noted. Medications tend to be given in somewhat higher dosages than in the outpatient setting because the dosages can be readjusted quickly. Residents are usually more confident about medication in the hospital setting because there are more professionals around to help the patient deal with side effects and to provide education and support. Residents are also better able to consult with their supervisors.

In addition, residents can arrange consultations with other physicians should there be worries about interactions with patients' other medical problems. Family meetings are usually organized to discuss a range of issues, and medications can be an item for discussion if the family and patient so choose. Moreover, the hospital usually has medications available in a wide range of preparations (e.g., pills, liquid, injection), so there are options if the patient has difficulty with one type of preparation. The pharmacists in the hospital are usually very helpful with cutting pills and making it as easy as possible for patients to receive medications that are ordered.

Outpatient

The outpatient setting is more difficult for the resident with regard to prescribing medications. For residents, the most significant difference between outpatient and inpatient settings is that supervision is usually less intense. In many outpatient settings, there is an attending psychiatrist who sits in for key portions of the initial evaluation of the patient and who may discuss initial impressions regarding medication. After the first session, however, the patient may often be seen by only the resident. The attending psychiatrist who first saw the patient may continue to supervise the case. Alternatively, depending on the form of psychotherapy provided to the patient (e.g., cognitive-behavioral therapy), someone who is well trained in that particular type of therapy might supervise the case instead. Thus, the primary supervision might be provided not by a psychiatrist but by a behavioral psychologist or an analyst. Supervision of the type of medication prescribed might be done by a general supervisor, who may be supervising the resident in his or her work with a number of patients. The resident might only discuss problem cases with the supervisor or might go over every case for a short amount of time. The resident may be quite independent about the type of medication chosen for patients and only bring up very particular issues with the supervisor.

Another complicating issue is that patients are frequently discharged after short inpatient hospitalizations even though they are only partially improved (frequently just after the issue of dangerousness is "resolved"). These patients are often discharged after their complex set of medications has been changed to another complex set of medications and while they are still dealing with numerous side effects. In this situation, the resident is expected to titrate patient medications down safely and help the patient to become functional again very quickly. This may not always be easy or possible. Additionally, the resident may face a complex set of medications that he or she does not agree with or is not well informed about (the preferences of inpatient and outpatient psychiatrists may be different). This situation may require more intense supervision in an environment where supervision is less available.

As opposed to inpatient units, where there is a steady and constant monitoring of medication issues, in the outpatient setting there is usually an interval of time between when the patient is first prescribed the medication and when the resident next sees the patient. The resident should inquire about the patient's form of payment for medication to make sure, for example, that the proposed medication will be on the patient's pharmacy formulary. Copayments are an issue, especially for many patients who are taking a number of medications. This is also a matter for discussion.

The resident might want to ask the patient to call and discuss how he or she is doing with the medication before the next appointment, especially if the follow-up appointment is not for a few weeks. The practice of scheduling a follow-up appointment for a new patient several weeks after the initial meeting should be discouraged—the patient should be seen frequently (e.g., within 1–2 weeks) during the initial phase of any treatment to help dispel anxieties about the treatment, side effects, and other issues and to foster the doctor–patient relationship. This approach to scheduling helps the resident find out about any negative side effects or problems that the patient might be having with the medication; allows the resident to discuss the dosage (and change it if necessary); and most importantly, enables the patient to feel that the resident cares about the impact of the medication and that the resident and the patient are in a partnership regarding medication.

Many patients may want to use e-mail to communicate with the resident, but we urge that communication regarding medication be conducted over the telephone and that such conversations be documented in the patient's chart. E-mails should also be documented in the chart—the best way is simply to copy the e-mail, which is especially easy in the case of the electronic medical record. There are various problems with e-mail communication (e.g., confidentiality, lack of non-verbal cues), and because there are so many potential problems with medication, we suggest that voice calls over the telephone be used instead of e-mail or texting (Silk and Yager 2003). Patients should be encouraged to call if any unpleasant side effects occur prior to their next appointment, and it should be emphasized that such a call is welcomed and is not a bother to the physician.

Because patients are usually working or are engaged in relationships in the outpatient setting, it is important to find out the impact that medications have on their jobs. For example, if the patient is driving as part of his or her job, does the psychotropic medication affect the patient's ability to drive or to have quick reflexes? If so, there may be a need to modify either the medication or the time of day it is taken, or to try to have the patient's work responsibilities changed.

Most psychotropic medications affect libido or have other sexual side effects, so it is important for the resident to ask the patient questions about these effects. Patients are often too embarrassed to raise such issues and feel more secure when the resident is asking about such important matters. The same is true for weight gain, sleep problems, and constipation, so these ideally would all be routine questions.

Sometimes patients will note that their significant other or various family members are concerned about the medication they are taking. It is helpful for the resident to understand this concern, because it could be a deterrent to the patient's adhering to the medication regimen. It could be useful, for example, to have the concerned family member attend part of a session or a full session with the patient to discuss any problems.

. Medication should be kept from young children. It is important for the resident to ascertain who at home might have access to the patient's medication and to make sure that the medication is kept in a safe and secure location. If the patient does not want the children to know about the psychiatric problems or the medication, the resident should discuss this matter with the patient.

Patients—and, in the case of children and adolescents, their parents—may be concerned about the possible association between antidepressants and suicidality (the so-called black box warning) that they may have seen on TV or read about. This relationship should be properly framed and discussed. Patients and family members should be asked to call immediately in the case of emergent suicidality. Children and adolescents should be monitored (seen) more frequently during the initial phase of treatment, as recommended by the U.S. Food and Drug Administration. Parents should be informed about the possibility (no matter how rare) of emergent suicidality, its frequent monitoring, and their ability to address it through questioning with their children. It is also important to actively ascertain the patient's suicidality, homicidality, and potential for violence prior to treatment and at every session, particularly when the patient is taking psychotropic medication.

Comorbid Medical Conditions and Substance Abuse/Dependence

Medical Conditions

Residents should be knowledgeable about their patients' medical conditions, what medications their patients are taking, and their patients' medical and surgical histories. Allergies to medications should be noted. Especially in the outpatient setting, the resident must let the patient know that changes in medical conditions or medications during the interval between appointments need to be reported to the resident.

Communication between the resident and the primary care providers or specialists should usually be done with the patient's written consent (although the Health Insurance Portability and Accountability Act [HIPAA] does not require such consent for communication among treating parties). It is imperative that residents let the other providers know when psychotropic medications are added or changed. Most patients are very appreciative that such communication occurs. Some patients will be embarrassed or say they will feel stigmatized if their primary care provider or other doctors know about their need for psychotropic medication. In such cases, there needs to be frank and open discussion between the resident and the patient, and the resident should point out that he or she cannot provide good care to the patient if such information is not provided to the other clinicians and that the rule of confidentiality does not apply in this communication. Serious harm to the patient could result if the other clinicians do not know about the patient's use of psychotropic medication. For example, there could be problems with interactions between medications; changes in blood concentrations of medications could occur if the various prescribers do not know about all the medications the patient is taking. If a patient prohibits such communication, the resident must seriously question whether proper care can be provided to the patient, and alternatives must be discussed.

The patient (and all physician and clinician providers) should be clear about who is in charge of what medications. Primary care physicians should not, for example, prescribe psychotropic medication or change dosages without letting the psychiatrist and other mental health clinicians know, and vice versa: the psychiatrist should not prescribe medications other than psychotropic medications (although there are emergency exceptions for both parties). If there is no electronic medical record or if the patient is not being seen in a closed system, the caregivers should discuss ahead of time how to transmit such information in a timely fashion (e.g., telephone, e-mail, fax, letter). It should not be the responsibility of the patient to be the provider of such information.

Substance Abuse/Dependence

Substance abuse and dependence are the subject of another important discussion, especially in the outpatient setting, where patients have greater access to substances with potential for abuse or dependence. Patients often do not like to admit their dependence on and use of substances such as nicotine, alcohol, marijuana, and other drugs. In addition, there are many patients who have dependences on prescribed medications such as hydrocodone bitartrate (Vicodin) and acetaminophen/oxycodone hydrochloride (Tylox). It is important for the resident not to make assumptions about such problems but rather to ask questions, make proper referrals for substance abuse treatment, and watch carefully if prescriptions for benzodiazepines, for example, are used up too quickly. Residents should actively ask whether patients are on any opioid painkillers, especially when prescription of a benzodiazepine is contemplated (these two classes of medications should not be prescribed together—another black box warning). If the resident discovers that the patient is already taking an opiate and a benzodiazepine, the patient must discontinue one of them; the resident may follow the example of pain medicine specialists who ask patients to make the choice of which of the two medications they would prefer to take. If patients are not doing as well as expected with a certain medication over a certain period of time, the resident should think about whether there may be a confounding substance problem. If patients are asking for medical leave that is not commensurate with the primary psychiatric diagnosis, then the resident should think about the possibility of substance abuse. It is important to obtain a good history of these types of problems when starting treatment and when prescribing psychotropic medication. The patient should continue to be assessed for ongoing problems.

It is also important to consider the role and influence of Alcoholics Anonymous (AA). Frequently, AA participants and sponsors (especially the less experienced ones) discourage patients from using psychotropic medications. They may be right in discouraging the use of benzodiazepines, but antidepressants (which some AA members call brain depressants) are wrongly stigmatized.

Other Conditions

Other disorders and conditions, such as personality disorders, history of trauma, and severe physical illness may impact the selection of medication and psychotherapy. For instance, supportive psychotherapy or interpersonal psychotherapy may be suited for patients with cancer, but some cancer medications may interact with psychotropic medications and so forth.

To summarize, the first encounter with the patient is one of the most difficult for the resident, especially in the outpatient setting. There are multiple issues to assess, but the key issue is the following:

Competency

At the initial outpatient session, psychiatry residents must demonstrate the ability to establish a doctor–patient relationship and to provide a trusting, warm environment to explore the patient's needs and problems. Psychiatry residents must be able to discuss medication properly and explain possible side effects and complications.

The resident ideally should determine, in the first session or two, what diagnosis to give the patient and, following from that, what type of treatment—psychotherapy, pharmacotherapy, both, neither, etc.—would be recommended.

Factors Affecting Psychotherapy Treatment Planning

- *Developing a formulation*—A biopsychosocial formulation is the key to understanding a patient's diagnosis and treatment plan. Many residents have difficulty with such formulations because they fall short on the "psych" part of the assessment. Often this has to do with not asking enough of the right questions during the interview. Furthermore, residents need to learn to develop hunches and offer these hunches to patients as a beginning point for discussion. This is a difficult skill to teach and hone because it is based on having experience, seeing a lot of patients, and reading case material—ingredients that are not generally available to a beginning resident.

- *Selecting the psychotherapy modality*—It is almost impossible to recommend a certain modality of psychotherapy without having experience providing it oneself, or having seen a supervisor or attending psychiatrist provide it, or having read about it. This is when supervision is very important, because the attending psychiatrist should step in and make a recommendation for the type of psychotherapy that might best work for the patient. It is difficult for residents to have to recommend a kind of treatment to a patient without having firsthand knowledge that it will work and benefit the patient. This is one of the aspects of medical care and education that makes residents want to hurry up and learn everything as soon as possible. Unfortunately, with various forms of psychotherapy, this is difficult for the beginning resident to do. Sometimes acknowledging such issues for residents under supervision is a good first step. Discussion of selecting a psychotherapy modality in a diagnostic conference with supervisors or in a similar venue can be crucial for the resident's selection of an appropriate psychotherapy modality.

- *Formulating the problem list*—Although the psychiatric diagnosis is determined by using the *Diagnostic and Statistical Manual of Mental Disorders* (DSM), psychiatrists function under the medical model whereby they must address the patient's issues in terms of a problem summary list. The patient's presenting problems are added to the list that already exists in the patient's file or electronic medical record. For the psychiatry resident, there are issues of confidentiality, privacy, and other matters that must be addressed in all systems of care. In addition, it is sometimes daunting for residents to publicly note a problem on a record that other attending physicians of other medical specialties can read. The problem summary list is something that needs to be addressed by the supervising attending psychiatrists and reviewed along with the resident's notes, charts, and so forth. What goes on the problems list and what comes off it are critically important parts of the patient's record.

- *Prioritizing problems*—It is important for the resident to first determine the list of problems and then, with the patient's help, determine how to prioritize and sequence these problems. This is difficult because it often requires discussing issues that are not necessarily clear to the patient (or to the clinician) at the time. Sometimes this requires waiting for further information or insight from other family members, waiting for a new job, waiting for a change in marital structure, or waiting for results of medical tests before determining the next steps. It is important for the resident to be patient and provide guidance without being intrusive and without moving too far ahead of the patient.

- *Determining treatment aims*—One of the major tasks for the resident and patient is to determine the aims—both pharmacological and psychotherapeutic—of the treatment. Once established, these aims should be constantly evaluated and reevaluated, as they may need to be modified or changed. Assumptions should be avoided in the process. This undertaking is challenging for a novice resident, however, and combining medication and psychotherapy makes it difficult to tease apart cause and effect. Nevertheless, this is a major task that should be addressed at every session and that should constitute part of the competency skills of the resident.

- *Explaining the selected psychotherapy modality*—Many patients view psychotherapy just as a free-talking cure and are not aware that they need to be very actively involved in some treatment modalities (e.g., cognitive-behavioral therapy) and may even have homework between sessions. The psychiatry resident should be able to explain why a particular modality was selected and what its structure and features are.

- *Outlining the time frame*—One of the questions most frequently asked by patients and their families is how long the process is going to take—how long will they need to take medication, and how long and how often do they need to receive psychotherapy? Patients and their families will want to know how soon patients will begin to feel better, how long it will take for the symptoms to improve, when they can go back to work, or when they can expect to start doing better at school. These are difficult but key concerns. An answer of "I don't know" from the resident could undermine the confidence that the patient has in the treatment process. Yet that may be the best answer the resident can give at the time. It is important for the resident to learn how to gauge the patient's level of distress and how much the patient is able to understand. Residents also need to learn the best way to explain the diagnosis and treatment plan and the best ways that the resident and patient can share with each other in the course of care and recovery.

Competency

During the evaluation phase, psychiatry residents must be able to demonstrate the ability to develop a biopsychosocial formulation of the patient's problems, develop a problem list, and, together with the patient, develop treatment aims and prioritize problems. Residents must be able to explain to the patient what treatment is being used and why the treatment is appropriate.

References

Beitman BD, Blinder BJ, Thase ME, et al: Integrating Psychotherapy and Pharmacotherapy. New York, WW Norton, 2003

Bender S, Messner E: Becoming a Therapist: What Do I Say, and Why? New York, Guilford, 2003

Bush FN, Sandberg LS: Combined treatment for depression. Psychiatr Clin N Am 35(1): 165–179, 2012

Carli T: The psychologically informed psychopharmacologist, in Psychopharmacology and Psychotherapy: A Collaborative Approach. Edited by Riba MB, Balon R. Washington, DC, American Psychiatric Press, 1999, pp 179–196

Colli A, Tanzilli A, Dimaggio G, et al: Patient personality and therapist response: an empirical investigation. Am J Psychiatry 171(1):102–108, 2014 24077643

Donkers T, Griffiths KM, Cuijpers P, et al: Psychoeducation for depression, anxiety and psychological distress: a meta-analysis. BMC Med 7:79, 2009 20015347

Hsiung RC (ed): E-Therapy: Case Studies, Guiding Principles, and the Clinical Potential of the Internet. New York, WW Norton, 2002

Keller MB, McCullough JP, Klein DN, et al: A comparison of nefazodone, the cognitive behavioral-analysis system of psychotherapy, and their combination for the treatment of chronic depression. N Engl J Med 342(20):1462–1470, 2000 10816183

Köhler S, Hoffmann S, Unger T, et al: Effectiveness of cognitive-behavioural therapy plus pharmacotherapy in inpatient treatment of depressive disorders. Clin Psychol Psychother 20(2):97–106, 2013 22095701

Nemeroff CB, Heim CM, Thase ME, et al: Differential responses to psychotherapy versus pharmacotherapy in patients with chronic forms of major depression and childhood trauma. Proc Natl Acad Sci U S A 100(24):14293–14296, 2003 14615578

Silk KR, Yager J: Suggested guidelines for e-mail communication in psychiatric practice. J Clin Psychiatry 64(7):799–806, 2003 12934981

Simon R: Unilateral treatment termination: "You're fired." Psychiatr Times, July, 2004, pp 25–26

Tasman A, Riba M, Silk K (eds): The Doctor-Patient Relationship in Pharmacotherapy: Improving Treatment Effectiveness. New York, Guilford, 2000

Evaluation and Opening in Integrated Treatment

3

The evaluation of every patient begins at the time of initial contact, whether that contact is with a physician, with a clinician performing a triage interview, or with a clinic staff member who is representing the doctor. The preliminary evaluation is focused on collecting the data that the clinician considers pertinent for making a diagnosis and determining the appropriate treatment. Del Piccolo and Goss (2012) have noted the importance of trying to understand the patient's problems and concerns even at this early stage of data gathering. This first interaction also serves as the beginning of the therapeutic alliance and as the moment when the patient may begin to partner with the health care team. This therapeutic encounter between the patient, who is the expert on his or her own experience and distress, and the psychiatrist, who can bring expertise to relieve suffering and restore health, is very important.

Because this chapter deals with integrated treatment (the resident providing both the psychotherapy and the medication or other medical care), we do not discuss the diagnosis of and decision making about patients who are referred to a psychiatrist for the sole purpose of treatment with medication or other medical treatment (e.g., electroconvulsive therapy). For example, there is a literature on comparing the effectiveness of integrated versus split/collaborative treatment for patients with severe personality disorder and/or those patients with suicidality and impulsivity (Bozzatello and Bellino 2016; Vaslamatzis et al. 2014). We will not focus on these special types of patients and symptom clusters in this chapter.

Instead, in this chapter, we discuss evaluating the patient and opening the treatment process (both psychopharmacology and psychotherapy), either with a new patient or with a patient who is referred to a psychiatrist after therapy with a nonphysician therapist. A referral may occur in the context of a patient newly in need of care, an established patient preferring a new arrangement, or the patient or therapist changing locations. A referral may occur because of nonprogression in treatment. We would like to emphasize that no matter what the situation (a patient who is being seen for the first time by someone or a patient who has been referred from someone else), the evaluation should be the same—thorough, detailed, and systematic so as not to forget important topics. Information should not be left unexplored simply because it was already obtained and provided by the referral source to the evaluating psychiatrist. Information from the referral source should be probed and rechecked with the patient. Accepting the interpretation of others could be misleading at times, whereas reinterpreting clinical data using newly collected information is generally useful and helpful. It may also be helpful, at some point, to explore with the patient what might have gone wrong in previous relationships with other therapists or psychiatrists in order to help the patient sort through what might be helpful, or not, going forward. With the consent of the patient, the resident may also decide to speak to the outside or former therapist/psychiatrist. This data-gathering step may impact how the resident thinks of the patient in terms of diagnosis, treatment adherence, and so forth, so the timing of this communication needs to be carefully thought out and, ideally, discussed in supervision.

It should be made clear to the patient during first contact that the initial session (or first few sessions) will be devoted to an evaluation and that any decision about treatment modality or modalities will occur only after the evaluation is completed. This helps the patient understand that the resident is not going to make a quick judgment. Instead, by seeing the patient over time, the resident will try to understand the complexity of the issues that the patient faces.

Bender and Messner (2003) suggest that framing the first session as a consultation or evaluation may have an important advantage. Both the patient and the psychiatrist can evaluate whether they are a good match and whether they feel comfortable working with each other. Both are given "the freedom to view the first meeting as an introduction without an obligation to continue" (Bender and Messner 2003, p. 17). Framing the first contact as a consultation is probably much easier in an outpatient setting. The concept of the first session (or sessions) being a consultation or evaluation may be also very useful in starting the treatment of children or adolescents. There are more parties involved, such as one or both parents, and finding a good match is therefore more complicated.

As in other clinical work, the initial step in the evaluation during integrated treatment is to establish an accurate diagnosis. It must be emphasized that although the diagnosis is an important element in treatment decision making, it is not the sole element. The diagnosis does not provide much information about the individual or about the individual's particular needs in treatment planning. There are other elements—such as the patient's previous response to treatment, symptoms (e.g., sleep disturbance, suicidality), cooperation or resistance, family history, support system, medical history, and value and belief systems—that may have a significant impact on treatment planning. An important and evolving area that should be taken into account in the evaluation and diagnosis is adversity and trauma, including childhood trauma, and how this shapes the patient's struggles. These issues may be culturally determined and will be important aspects of the integrated biopsychosocial approach that is needed to carefully explore the patient's subjective psychological experience (Brenner 2016). Thus, information about these and other factors should be gathered in the first session (or sessions) to help inform the decision about treatment.

First Contact: Technical Remarks

The first contact between the psychiatrist and the patient usually starts in the waiting area. In some clinics, as part of the intake process, the patient might have been screened for depression, anxiety, and other psychiatric conditions using scales such as nine-item Patient Health Questionnaire (PHQ-9) and the Generalized Anxiety Disorder (GAD) test, either on paper or on a computer. After being triaged and being given an appointment, the patient arrives full of various expectations and curious about the results of the questionnaires that were filled out. The patient may be wondering, "Who is this doctor? What will I be asked? Are we going to get along?" Some patients may be worried that they will be committed to a hospital setting. Others may be worried about the stigma they might face if others find out where they are. In this era of increased concerns about confidentiality, the psychiatrist needs to make sure that the patient's identity is protected. Calling the patient by last name in the waiting area might be problematic because it reveals the patient's identity. The psychiatrist can call the patient by first name; however, that may not sit well with some patients, particularly older patients. Many experts (e.g., Bender and Messner 2003) advise psychiatrists to simply identify the patient who is waiting, approach the patient, ask whether he or she is waiting to see this particular psychiatrist, and then invite the patient to follow or come in. Some clinics have specific protocols about this and even use a beeper system to identify patients.

After taking the patient to the office and making him or her as comfortable as possible—for example, by asking the patient to take off his or her coat—the resident should explain what is going to happen during the first session or two. It should be made clear approximately how long the session is going to last and what is expected to come out of it. In addition, the resident should explain who will have access to the patient's medical record and if other doctors will be able to read the psychiatric notes. Residents should remember that the formation of the therapeutic alliance begins at this time. As Bender and Messner (2003, p. 29) point out, the therapist should be responsive and not overbearing and should be careful not to underdirect or overdirect the first session. As Del Piccolo and Goss (2012) note, patients should feel, from the very beginning, that their contributions are essential for diagnostic and treatment planning. A more interactive model and partnership between patient and resident is optimal (Edwards and Elwyn 2009; Evans et al. 2003).

The resident should be observant of the patient's behavior during this period: does the patient seem anxious, avoid making eye contact, wring his or her hands, have tremors, or sit at the edge of the chair? It is also polite, appropriate, and practical to inform the patient that confidential notes will be taken during the information-gathering session if this is the case. The patient's feelings about the psychiatrist's note taking during the session should also be explored. As MacKinnon and Yudofsky (1991, p. 10) note, some patients may resent the psychiatrist for *not* taking notes during the interview, because it would make them feel that what they said was not sufficiently important or that the doctor was uninterested. Other patients, as MacKinnon and Yudofsky also note, cannot tolerate note taking because they feel that it distracts the psychiatrist's attention from them.

It is important to make sure that writing information down does not become the dominant activity of the information-gathering session. One should write basic information and scribble down the most important data without interrupting the flow of the interview and without avoiding eye contact with the patient. There may also be times during the interview when the interviewer should stop taking notes, putting the pen and paper or the laptop down. This applies to situations when intimate or sensitive issues, such as sexual issues or negative feelings about any previous treatment, are discussed (MacKinnon and Yudofsky 1991).

In these times when nearly everything is computerized, many psychiatrists are switching to electronic medical records. In fact, some institutions encourage note taking done directly on the computer or laptop, which encourages efficiency but may have an impact on making eye contact and forging an alliance. The same rules applicable to writing on paper apply to typing electronic notes. We advise psychiatrists not to type into the computer during the session (although we have heard of and have witnessed nonpsychiatrist physicians doing so). Instead, paper notes could be transferred to the computer after the session. It is advisable to transcribe or type notes *right after* seeing the patient instead of waiting until the end of a busy day, when the memories of several patient histories could merge and facts could get confused. (We have also witnessed nonpsychiatrist physicians dictating notes in front of patients, which is not recommended.)

Many psychiatrists start the initial evaluation by obtaining basic patient data such as age, marital status, and employment. Others advocate beginning the session with an open-ended question such as "Why are you coming to see me?"; "What can I do for you?"; or "How can I help you?" The patient should be left to answer these questions without interruption if possible (although manic or psychotic patients may have to be interrupted). The resident should acknowledge that he or she is listening by occasionally making comments or sounds such as "Hmm" or "Interesting." The patient should be asked to provide more details whenever possible and appropriate. The psychiatrist should encourage the patient by making comments such as "Tell me more about this" whenever necessary. One should also think and frame questions in terms such as "Why now; why is the patient coming to see me and telling me this at this point in his or her life?" Since this is a partnership between the psychiatrist and the patient, the patient should, it is hoped, become curious about the questions and answers; this forms "the hook" in helping to forge ahead.

Although we discuss information gathering in a certain structural fashion, progressing from the chief complaint and present illness through various parts of the history to the mental status examination, it is important to realize that 1) various parts of the examination overlap (e.g., present illness and parts of the mental status examination); 2) the sequence of the patient evaluation is not etched in stone—flexibility is key; and 3) the resident should not avoid following cues for the sake of keeping a rigid information-gathering outline. One mistake that is frequently made by beginning clinicians is putting aside certain matters that are seemingly unrelated to the questions asked. This decision could lead to a very important therapeutic issue being missed and could also make the patient feel that the resident is not really interested in the patient's concerns. An example of a psychiatrist missing a cue is a situation in which a patient responds to the opening question "What is bringing you here?" by saying, with her eyes full of tears, "I am a widow." A response by the inexperienced resident would be, "OK, but why are you here now?"

Sometimes, residents worry that the attending physician or supervisor will be angry that not enough information was obtained, and this worry overwhelms the entire evaluation. We understand this and suggest that the resident and attending physician or supervisor discuss this issue.

The initial evaluation is usually finished in a preliminary form within the first hour or so designated for the assessment. Evaluation of an inpatient (except in the emergency department) may require more time. Often, even the most experienced clinician may not be able to finish the initial evaluation and establish a preliminary diagnosis within the time frame of the first contact, and a subsequent evaluation session may have to be scheduled. In addition, the resident needs to evaluate the patient over time, whether in the inpatient or outpatient setting, so that the resident does not arrive at prematurely a diagnosis that does not adequately capture the complexity of the patient's concerns. Most initial evaluations of adult patients are simply evaluations of the patient himself or herself. However, in some cases, evaluations may involve the interview of relatives or significant others. An evaluation of a child or adolescent should always, if possible, include an interview with parents or guardians (together with the child and also separately).

Initial Evaluation Outline

It is important to note that the order of various parts of the initial evaluation may be a matter of personal preference or custom. Furthermore, there may be templates in the medical record that are standardized. However, after obtaining basic identifying data, the resident should start with the inquiry about the chief complaint and present illness. (For a more thorough review of the American Psychiatric Association's Practice Guidelines for the Psychiatric Treatment of Adults, see Silverman et al. 2015.)

Chief Complaint and Present Illness

Even though the chief complaint is traditionally listed on outlines and templates of psychiatric evaluations, it is not something the resident must always ask about, but it is something he or she identifies in the written summary of the examination. The chief complaint could be a direct quote of the patient's response to the question "How can I help you?" or "Why do you think you need help?" Or it could be a very brief, simple summary of the patient's main complaint ("Patient has been depressed for the past 3 weeks," or "Sudden onset of panic attacks 3 weeks ago"). It may also serve as an introduction to the next part of the evaluation, the present illness. The patient's general medical status and recent health should be assessed thoroughly, especially for sudden-onset mental health concerns, as part of the exploration of the history of present illness.

The questioning about the history of the present illness should start with open-ended questions. The questioning usually becomes more direct and targeted through the interview. Depending on the clinical situation, broad questions should be replaced by focused or targeted questions about the symptoms, their onset, possible precipitating factors, impact on functioning, the scope of distress, maladaptive patterns, and other issues. Some patients may be able to provide a fairly chronological account of their present illness. Others may need to be asked specific questions about the onset and other clinical factors. Depending on the clinical material provided by the patient, answers to questions asked by the resident may later help in the selection of treatment (medication, psychotherapy, or both).

It may not always be possible to clearly separate the history of the present illness from the past psychiatric history or history of previous psychiatric illnesses. An example is the case of recurrent major depression. The most recent episode of depression may represent the present illness, but it should not be totally separated from previous episodes of depression.

The history of the present illness could include what some call the "psychiatric review of systems" (MacKinnon and Yudofsky 1991). This review includes questions about the patient's sleep pattern, appetite, weight regulation, bowel functioning, and sexual functioning (MacKinnon and Yudofsky 1991). Assessment of suicidality should also be included in this part of the evaluation. Assessment of suicidality could begin with broader questions such as asking whether the patient has been feeling that life is not worth living. The assessment of suicidality and homicidality, however, should ultimately be specific and well documented. (Does the patient have vague suicidal ideation or a specific plan? If the patient has a plan, is the selected modality available? What is the overall risk? Is a safety net available? Does the patient own a gun/guns? Where are the guns stored? Are they locked?) Some clinics use standardized screening tools and guidelines for suicidality to help with consistency and training of residents (American Psychiatric Association 2003).

The interviewer should not remain focused on only one area of the problem and psychopathology. After establishing a very preliminary possible diagnosis, the resident should always probe other areas of psychopathology (e.g., in depressed patients, the resident should ask about anxiety, psychosis, and so forth).

Psychiatric and Medical Illness History

The patient's personal history of psychiatric illness is a very important component of the initial evaluation. Such a history could have a tremendous impact on treatment planning and selection of treatment modality. A patient with a recent episode of major depression and a history of two previous episodes of major depression should probably start lifelong treatment of this illness. The suicidality of a patient with a history of several serious suicide attempts should be viewed differently than a suicidal gesture in a patient with no previous history of suicidality. A positive response to previous treatment should guide the resident to use the same treatment again and vice versa.

The patient should be probed about onset of past illness, possible precipitating factors, course, comorbidity, accompanying disability, and treatment. As noted above under "Chief Complaint and Present Illness," at times it is difficult to separate the history of the present illness from the overall psychiatric illness history. Information about psychiatric hospitalizations should include the patient's age at the time of hospitalization, reason for hospitalization, length of hospitalization, place of hospitalization (the psychiatrist may or may not be familiar with the place and may need to obtain records from the hospital), what was done during the hospitalization (medications tried, psychotherapy), response to treatment, possible side effects, feelings about the treatment, the patient's condition at discharge, and the patient's feelings about the hospitalization.

The patient should be asked about details of past treatment. Questions about medications should include the names of the medications, the patient's understanding of the reasons a particular medication was used, the length of treatment with each particular medication, maximum dosages, whether the medication was helpful, which symptoms were relieved the most, and what side effects were present. Questions about medication allergies should be also asked, but the resident should make a distinction between true allergy and a serious side effect. Many psychotic patients will frequently say that they are allergic to one of the antipsychotics. Detailed questioning may reveal that they had a dystonic reaction when taking a higher dosage. The patient should also be asked whether he or she is taking any psychotropic medication at the time of the initial evaluation. As Bender and Messner (2003) emphasize, residents should not assume that the patient is not taking psychotropic medication if he or she is not seeing a psychiatrist, as many primary care physicians prescribe psychotropic medications. Many primary care physicians are even mandated by managed care companies to try psychotropic medication and to refer the patient to a psychiatrist only after the first treatment attempt fails. The patient should be asked about previous psychotherapy and behavioral therapy (i.e., when, why, what kind, success/failure, patient's feelings about the treatment). The resident should also ask the patient whether medication was combined with psychotherapy or behavioral therapy in the past.

Previous suicidal and homicidal thoughts and behavior should be explored and documented (age at the time of suicide attempt, relationship to symptoms, planned or impulsive attempt, modality used, feelings about death at the time of the suicide attempt, whether it was a suicidal gesture, subsequent treatment, and the patient's current feelings about a particular suicide attempt). It is also important to make a distinction between suicidal and self-harming or self-mutilating behavior. In addition, any time spent in jail or prison should be reviewed and documented thoroughly.

A thorough exploration of possible substance abuse history, including smoking, may be part of the overall psychiatric history or part of the personal and social history. The patient should be asked about substances used or abused, age at commencement of substance abuse, duration (if not continuous), frequency, amount used, money spent on the substance abused, how the substance was obtained, possible association with illegal activities (e.g., selling drugs), complications (medical [e.g., hepatitis, AIDS]; psychiatric [e.g., depression, withdrawal, blackouts]; relational; financial; employment-related), immediate effect of the substance abused (feeling better, improved mood, relief of anxiety), personal feelings about substance abuse (feelings of guilt or shame), situations in which the substance abuse occurred (alone, with a group), and previous treatment and its results (inpatient, outpatient). Because marijuana has been legalized in some U.S. states and, as of 2017, 28 states and the District of Columbia allow the use of medical marijuana, patients should be asked specifically about marijuana use, as they may not consider it worth mentioning. Similar questions should be asked specifically about alcohol use. Patients should also be questioned about tobacco (smoking or chewing, and how much) and caffeine use (the number cups of coffee a day, the amount of other caffeinated beverages).

Medical history is an important part of the psychiatric evaluation. The history of serious illnesses, especially chronic ones, and surgeries should be obtained. The resident should consider whether the symptoms with which the patient presents are either a manifestation of the chronic illness or a reaction to the chronic illness, or whether the symptoms are not related to the illness. Specific questions should also be asked to determine the possibility of a seizure disorder or head injury. The patient should also be asked about medications used to treat any medical conditions. Preferably, the patient should provide a list of these medications and dosages. Many medications can induce various symptoms—such as depression, anxiety, and fatigue—and thus mimic mental disorders. Many medications can also interfere with the metabolism of psychotropic agents.

Female patients should always be asked about their menstrual history, including the age at menarche, regularity of cycle, possible menopause (depending on age), use of contraceptives, and symptoms associated with menstruation (e.g., pain, cramping, changes of mood, irritability), including the possible alleviation of these symptoms with hormones and medications (e.g., antidepressants). Before medication is started, women of childbearing age should be asked about the possibility of pregnancy, and possibly get tested.

The medical history should include a brief review of systems; many institutional templates require this for both inpatient and outpatient assessments. The resident can ask the patient, "Is there anything that I left out or should have asked? Is there something important that I should have asked?" This gives the patient an opportunity to add something and also reminds the resident that perhaps something was missed.

Family History

Information about a family history of psychiatric illness and family responses to treatment could also have an impact on treatment selection and planning.

Family history should include the family history of psychiatric and medical illness and explore the relationships within the family. Information about both parents should include their ages, if living (or age at the time of death and cause of death), history of mental disorders, history of medical illnesses, medications used to treat any psychiatric illnesses, and responses to medications. Information about siblings should include their ages (and the patient's birth order), presence of psychiatric illnesses, treatments, and responses to treatments. A history of psychiatric illness and treatment in members of the extended family (grandparents, aunts, uncles, cousins) should also be obtained. Besides asking about mental illness, we recommend asking specifically about substance abuse and history of suicide in family members. Many people do not think about substance abuse or suicide in terms of mental illness. One should also explore the relationships within the family, including how the patient gets along with his or her parents and siblings, whether there has been any violence within the family, and whether any abuse (physical or sexual) has occurred.

Asking about family history of medical illness may reveal interesting and important information—for example, a strong family history of hypothyroidism may reveal a possible diagnosis of this disease in a mildly depressed, tired patient.

Personal and Social History

Personal and social history is what makes the psychiatric evaluation different from an ordinary medical evaluation. Physicians in other disciplines may ask about parts of the personal history, but they do not usually obtain the personal and social history in entirety. This part of the evaluation may help the examining physician, in partnership with the family, determine optimal treatment planning in terms of the patient's preferences, family and social support, financial situation, and other factors. The personal and social history encompasses several areas; the clinician should attempt to elicit a full picture of the patient and his or her life situation, stressors, functional status, and goals. More and more appreciation is being given to *epigenetics*, the interaction of environmental influence and gene expression. Although we may not understand all the variables that induce epigenetic changes, it is probably a good idea for residents to think about the molecular biology of epigenetics and how new developments might impact usual forms of care, especially when exploring the patient's social history (Brenner 2016).

The personal history may start with the *perinatal and developmental history*. Information about the prenatal situation (e.g., family constellation, whether the parents wanted and planned to have a child, possible complications of pregnancy) and the patient's birth (e.g., premature, uncomplicated, forceps delivery, cesarean section, jaundice at birth, defect at birth) should be obtained. Many pieces of information that some recommend gathering—such as the parents' reaction to the patient's gender and selection of the patient's name (MacKinnon and Yudofsky 1991)—might not be realistically obtainable under the ever-present time pressure. Some residents, however, may have the luxury of having enough time to obtain this kind of information. Further information about personal history should include, if time and situation permit, developmental milestones, relationships during childhood and adolescence, and emerging personality (e.g., shy, defiant, oppositional) during childhood and adolescence.

Educational history should include information regarding whether the patient graduated from high school (if not, why not and whether a GED [General Educational Development diploma] was obtained), college education, postgraduate education (vs. current employment), and the patient's original educational goals and their fulfillment. The patient should be asked about any history of difficulties at school, either academic or behavioral. Educational level can have an impact on treatment adherence (Nosé et al. 2003).

Occupational history should include, if possible, information about all employment, including duration, reason for termination or change, any difficulties at work, and possible exposure to dangerous substances. An important question to consider is whether the patient's employment is commensurate with his or her education level. It is also important to understand if the patient's treatment goals include a change or improvement in occupation or quality of life (Kamenov et al. 2017).

Military history should include the age when the patient was drafted or recruited, reasons for signing up (e.g., idealism, financial reasons, or risk and thrill seeking), length of service, deployment, and the nature of and reason for discharge. Military history should also include information about whether the patient experienced combat, sustained any injuries, underwent any disciplinary actions, or was exposed to addictive and/or toxic substances during service. The resident should also ask what it was like returning home, the impact of the patient's service on family, and so forth.

Relational and marital history should include information about any sustained relationships in the patient's life. Inquiry should be made about the age when the patient got married, length of marriage or relationship, past conflicts and disagreements, and present relationship with the partner or spouse. If the patient is divorced, the reasons for divorce should be discussed. Information about children—their ages, health, education, and patient's relationship with them—should also be gathered. When the patient presents relational or marital issues as the core of his or her problems, the relational and marital history can be expanded by asking about areas of disagreement, who does what at home, the management of family finances, and relationships with members of the extended family.

Sexual history should include information about psychosexual development, early sexuality, sexual orientation, age at first sexual contact or intercourse, frequency of sexual activity, ability to reach orgasm, any sexual dysfunction (e.g., low libido, erectile dysfunction, lack of lubrication, premature ejaculation, delayed orgasm, anorgasmia, painful orgasm), masturbation, and unusual sexual preferences. We have noted that psychiatric residents frequently omit the sexual history for various reasons, either because they are uncomfortable asking patients about sex or because they are inappropriately worried about offending patients by asking about sexual history. We would like to emphasize that when asked tactfully and in full confidentiality, patients do not usually feel offended by questions about their sexuality and, in fact, appreciate that someone is taking the time to ask about this often-neglected subject.

Some (e.g., MacKinnon and Yudofsky 1991) also suggest asking about *social relationships, friends, religious and cultural background, hobbies, and long-term plans as a part of personal history*. Others (e.g., Bender and Messner 2003, p. 66) recommend obtaining an "adaptive history" by asking questions such as "What stresses have you overcome in the past?"; "How did you do it?"; "What are your personal strengths?"

Cultural history should focus on country of origin, where parents and grandparents are from, and how mental illness is viewed by the patient and the family. Unfortunately, in some cultures, having a mental illness, seeing a psychiatrist, and taking medications are still stigmatized, and it is helpful to understand this. Cultural standards also change over time. Brenner (2016) gives a good example of how bullying used to be viewed as a schoolyard problem that was painful but not necessarily toxic. Culturally, we now view bullying as a serious trauma that can increase the risk of suicide and contribute to later serious mental illness (Arseneault et al. 2010). Cultural standards toward mental illness may also change over time.

Mental Status Examination

The mental status examination is a summary of the physician's observations and the patient's subjective reporting of areas such as appearance, behavior, feelings, perception, thinking, and cognitive functioning. Most textbooks describe the mental status examination as a long list of categories to be examined at the end of the psychiatric evaluation. An experienced clinician, however, usually begins the mental status examination from the very beginning of the evaluation by observing the patient's appearance and behavior and registering the symptoms that the patient reports. The more formal mental status examination conducted at the end of the psychiatric evaluation should therefore address only areas not previously covered or areas in need of further clarification, such as specific cognitive assessments. The resident should not repeat detailed questioning about symptoms of major depression in a patient who presented with a chief complaint of depressed mood, low energy, poor sleep, and lack of appetite. Instead, the resident might ask about symptoms not mentioned before, such as anhedonia or cognitive impairment.

The mental status examination should include but not be limited to the following areas:

- *Attitude and rapport*—Whether the patient comes into the office voluntarily or hesitantly; whether the patient is cooperative, friendly, and appropriate; whether he or she makes eye contact; and the nature of the patient's facial expression.
- *Appearance*—The patient's hygiene, clothing, and special marks (e.g., tattoos).
- *Behavior and psychomotor activity*—The nature of the patient's gait; whether he or she is restless, sits on the edge of the chair, is wringing his or her hands, has increased motor activity; whether the patient has abnormal movements, tics, dystonias, gesticulations, and so forth. Some are now including this information in the review of systems in the electronic medical record template.
- *Speech*—The quantity (e.g., talking all the time or answering only in monosyllabic words) and quality (e.g., errors, tone, rate of production, rhythm) of the patient's speech.
- *Affect*—The expression on the patient's face.
- *Mood and mood congruence/appropriateness and stability (vs. lability)*— "Vegetative" signs, such as sleep (including dreams), appetite, and libido, should be explored. Exploration of this area should also include other symptoms of mood disorders, such as possible anhedonia, energy level, and feelings of guilt. The resident should ask about recent suicidal or homicidal ideation and possible plans.
- *Anxiety and related symptoms*—Obsessions, compulsions, panic attacks, worrying, social avoidance, phobias, flashbacks, and startle responses.
- *Perception*—Illusions, hallucinations, and feelings of unreality and depersonalization.
- *Thought process*—Form (e.g., flow of associations, blocking, tangentiality, circumstantiality) and content (e.g., suspiciousness, ideas of reference, thought insertion, delusions—systematized, vague, or isolated—and their content—paranoid or grandiose) of the patient's thought processes; also, in the case of mood disorders, congruency with mood.
- *Alertness and wakefulness.*
- *Orientation*—By time, place, person, and situation.
- *Concentration*—Tested by simple tasks such as serial sevens or spelling certain words forward and backward.
- *Memory*—Recent, intermediate, remote, possible confabulation. Short-term memory and concentration could be tested by asking the patient to remember three things and then asking him or her to recall these things in 5 minutes. (We have observed that many residents do not allow enough time between asking the patient to remember three things and asking for their recollection—asking for recollection almost immediately is meaningless.)

- *Estimate of general information and fund of knowledge*—The patient's ability to provide information about recent events, big cities, famous people, or geography.
- *Estimate of intelligence*—Average, below average, above average; or possible developmental delays.
- *Judgment*—Operational and formal; estimated by asking about reactions to standard situations.
- *Abstraction*—The patient's ability to abstract, which could be tested by asking him or her to interpret proverbs or by discussing similarities and differences.
- *Insight*—The patient's awareness of his or her illness or situation.
- *Impulse control and frustration tolerance.*

Formulation

After finishing the evaluation, the examining resident may briefly formulate the case, considering the key issues such as the patient's present illness, past illness, personal history, developmental issues, and ego strengths and defenses. The formulation may be postponed, however, until further information is gathered and any test results have been obtained.

Diagnosis

Making the diagnosis (or diagnoses) of the patient by using the multiaxial DSM diagnostic classification (DSM-IV-TR; American Psychiatric Association 2000) has been abandoned in the latest edition of DSM (DSM-5; American Psychiatric Association 2013). Many considered the multiaxial diagnosis cumbersome and insufficiently inclusive and considered Axis IV and DSM-IV-TR vague and not very useful. However, we believe that multiaxial diagnosis forces the clinician to consider various areas that may have an impact on treatment planning and treatment outcome, including diagnosis of major mental disorder; possible personality disorder or its traits; intellectual impairment; the presence of physical illness that might be involved in the pathogenesis and that might possibly complicate the treatment planning and outcome; the presence of major stressors; and the level of functioning.

Diagnostic considerations might include decisions about further medical testing, such as a physical examination, laboratory testing (either exploratory, such as thyroid testing for unexplained tiredness and low energy, or as a baseline before starting certain medications, such as liver enzyme testing before beginning certain antipsychotic medications or blood urea nitrogen, creatinine, and thyroid tests before starting lithium), measurement of heart rate and blood pressure before starting medications, possible psychological testing (e.g., memory and other cognitive testing), and neurological examination and other specialized diagnostic testing.

Competency

Psychiatry residents should, based on their evaluation of the patient and their preliminary diagnosis, be able to select the appropriate pharmacotherapy or psychotherapy, or combination.

Treatment Planning

The entire initial evaluation is focused on establishing the diagnosis, selecting the most appropriate treatment, and starting to develop the relationship or therapeutic alliance with the patient (Del Piccolo and Goss 2012). Both the diagnosis and the treatment selection and plan should be thoroughly discussed with the patient at the end of the initial evaluation (see "Discussion With the Patient/ Opening" below). The treatment selection is a very complicated process that includes the following (in no particular order of importance and not exclusively):

- Diagnosis
- Comorbidity
- Evidence-based medicine data
- Possible use of guidelines
- Consideration of target symptoms
- Previous treatment experience (both efficacy and side effects)
- Dangerousness (suicidality, homicidality)
- The patient's beliefs, possible illness denial, preferences, misconceptions, and expectations
- The patient's level of functioning and impairment
- The patient's personality traits or personality disorder
- Possible nonadherence to the medication regimen
- Possible involvement of another specialist (e.g., a nutritionist in the case of an eating disorder)
- Psychodynamic issues
- Consideration of possible side effects
- The physician's experience and skills
- Formation of the therapeutic alliance
- Cost of treatment
- Insurance regulations
- Availability of both patient and treating physician
- Physical location of treatment (inpatient, day treatment, outpatient)
- Existence of a support network

- Market seductions and pressures (on both physician and patient, such as those produced by direct-to-consumer advertisement)

Bender and Messner (2003) suggest organizing psychiatric diagnoses into two categories: 1) disorders with targetable symptoms that meet DSM diagnostic criteria (e.g., mood disorders, anxiety disorders, substance abuse) and 2) conditions more closely linked to ongoing life stressors (e.g., relational problems, occupational problems, adjustment disorders, personality disorders). This distinction may help the resident to make the decision about medication versus psychotherapy. Psychotherapy, however, is usually indicated in both categories, and medication could be indicated in either category or both categories. In many instances, the impairment of daily functioning may be a major factor in choosing medication. For instance, the physician may recommend starting cognitive-behavioral therapy in the case of major depressive disorder with mild or no functional impairment; however, he or she will recommend an antidepressant plus cognitive-behavioral therapy in the case of major depressive disorder with severe functional impairment. The decision as to which type of psychotherapy to select could be based on therapist training (whatever psychotherapy is the therapist's area of expertise), diagnosis (e.g., cognitive-behavioral therapy for depression or in vivo desensitization for agoraphobia without a history of panic attacks), or outcome (whatever the goal of therapy is, whatever could be realistically achieved [Makover 2016]). Assuming that the evaluating psychiatry resident is competent in various psychotherapies, decision making at the beginning of integrated treatment is going to have a diagnosis-based and outcome-based approach. For example, in a case of major depressive disorder, after considering numerous factors and selecting the most appropriate antidepressant, the psychiatrist may consider the diagnosis and immediate goals in selecting cognitive-behavioral therapy.

Competency

Psychiatry residents should be able to discuss with and explain to the patient the selection of treatment modalities and their rationale.

Discussion With the Patient/Opening

Discussing the diagnosis and the treatment selection and plan with the patient is usually the last step of the initial evaluation (unless the evaluation needs to be extended beyond the first session).

The patient should be informed, in simple terms, about the diagnosis and what the diagnosis means in practical terms. The patient should be encouraged to ask questions about the diagnosis and the diagnostic process. Interestingly, many patients are quite relieved once the diagnosis is made and they have a term—a symbolic explanation—for their problems.

After discussing the diagnosis, the resident should briefly outline the recommendation for the initial treatment plan. The resident should explain the selection of both the medication and psychotherapy, what to expect of each modality, the time frame (e.g., fairly quick alleviation of anxiety with benzodiazepines vs. 3 weeks waiting for an antidepressant to alleviate depressed mood), and possible side effects and their management. The patient should be also given instructions on how to reach the resident in case there is an emergency or if the patient experiences any bothersome side effects or has any questions. Patients especially appreciate the possibility of such contact, and the availability of the resident often alleviates a lot of their anxiety about starting treatment. As with the diagnosis, patients should be encouraged to ask questions about the treatment. Many patients may have very specific questions based on Internet searches, direct-to-consumer advertisement, or media reports or sensationalism. Finally, the patient should be given a follow-up appointment fairly soon (it is simply not acceptable to say, "Here is your prescription; see me in month or two"). Patients should be seen fairly frequently during the initial phase of any treatment.

As Beitman and colleagues (2003, p. 38) explain, the initiation of treatment should also include summarizing the patient's conceptualization of the illness and expectations of treatment, predicting possible side effects of pharmacotherapy, acknowledging negative treatment experiences, addressing the patient's denial of illness or need for treatment with inquiry into negative social consequences or lifestyle, and, in the case of pharmacotherapy, comparing mental illness and psychopharmacology to other medical problems and medications such as diabetes and insulin.

The issues of the cost or copay of medications and the ability to visit the clinic should also be raised to see if there are any barriers, such as transportation problems. These are practical matters that might impact seeing the patient or having the patient be able to take the prescribed medication. Sometimes patients are embarrassed to bring up costs, and it is helpful when the clinician can discuss the issue in a caring and empathic manner to see if some of the barriers can be addressed together.

In subsequent sessions during the opening phase of treatment, the resident may further deal with issues such as the meaning of medication for the patient, fear of addiction to medication, loss of control over behavior, loss of personality, confusion of symptoms and side effects, the natural tendency to stop treatment when symptoms improve, and benefits and drawbacks of treatment (Beitman et al. 2003).

Once the initial evaluation—in one or more sessions—is completed, all information is gathered, and various treatment issues mentioned in this chapter are considered, the resident should discuss the case with the clinical supervisor. The discussion of the diagnosis should include consideration of the impact of the diagnosis on treatment selection and, in the case of integrated or combined treatment, on the sequencing of treatment modalities.

Once the psychiatrist decides to initiate integrated treatment, he or she has to make a decision about sequencing pharmacotherapy and psychotherapy (which one to start first or whether to start both at the same time). Sequencing in integrated treatment is discussed in Chapter 4.

References

American Psychiatric Association: Diagnostic and Statistical Manual of Mental Disorders, 4th Edition, Text Revision. Washington, DC, American Psychiatric Association, 2000

American Psychiatric Association: Practice guideline for the assessment and treatment of patients with suicidal behaviors. Am J Psychiatry 160(11)(suppl):1–60, 2003 14649920

American Psychiatric Association: Diagnostic and Statistical Manual of Mental Disorders, 5th Edition. Arlington, VA, American Psychiatric Association, 2013

Arseneault L, Bowes L, Shakoor S: Bullying victimization in youths and mental health problems: 'much ado about nothing'? Psychol Med 40(5):717–729, 2010 19785920

Beitman BD, Blinder BJ, Thase ME, et al: Integrating Psychotherapy and Pharmacotherapy: Dissolving the Mind-Brain Barrier. New York, WW Norton, 2003

Bender S, Messner E: Becoming a Therapist: What Do I Say, and Why? New York, Guilford, 2003

Bozzatello P, Bellino S: Combined therapy with interpersonal psychotherapy adapted for borderline personality disorder: A two-years follow-up. Psychiatry Res 240:151–156, 2016 27107668

Brenner AM: Revisiting the biopsychosocial formulation: neuroscience, social science, and the patient's subjective experience. Acad Psychiatry 40(5):740–746, 2016 27060094

Del Piccolo L, Goss C: People-centred care: new research needs and methods in doctor-patient communication: challenges in mental health. Epidemiol Psychiatr Sci 21(2):145–149, 2012 22789161

Edwards A, Elwyn G: Shared Decision-Making: Achieving Evidence-Based Patient Choice. New York, Oxford University Press, 2009

Evans R, Edwards A, Elwyn G: The future for primary care: increased choice for patients. Qual Saf Health Care 12(2):83–84, 2003 12679499

Kamenov K, Twomey C, Cabello M, et al: The efficacy of psychotherapy, pharmacotherapy and their combination on functioning and quality of life in depression: a meta-analysis. Psychol Med 47(3):414–425, 2017 27780478

MacKinnon RA, Yudofsky SC: Principles of the Psychiatric Evaluation. Philadelphia, PA, JB Lippincott, 1991

Makover RB: Treatment Planning for Psychotherapists: A Practical Guide to Better Outcomes, 3rd Edition. Washington, DC, American Psychiatric Publishing, 2016

Nosé M, Barbui C, Gray R, et al: Clinical interventions for treatment non-adherence in psychosis: meta-analysis. Br J Psychiatry 183:197–206, 2003 12948991

Silverman JJ, Galanter M, Jackson-Triche M, et al; American Psychiatric Association: The American Psychiatric Association Practice Guidelines for the Psychiatric Evaluation of Adults. Am J Psychiatry 172(8):798–802, 2015 26234607

Vaslamatzis G, Theodoropoulos P, Vondikaki S, et al: Is the residential combined (psychotherapy plus medication) treatment of patients with severe personality disorder effective in terms of suicidality and impulsivity? J Nerv Ment Dis 202(2):138–143, 2014 24469526

Sequencing in Integrated Treatment

4

One of the most difficult issues for any psychiatrist—either a seasoned clinician or an early resident—is to determine a treatment plan based on a good working diagnosis. Developing a treatment plan in partnership with the patient that the patient can reasonably adhere to, that is based on realistic expectations for treating the patient's illness in a timely manner, and that is financially affordable for the patient is surely the goal. Some would say, however, that this is a combination of art and science. Others might argue that the development of treatment plans should be protocol or guideline driven. Still others might counter that there are so many factors to be weighed in a realistic treatment plan that it would be difficult to regulate something so individualistically driven.

Residents will probably combine medication with various therapy modalities, with supportive and cognitive-behavioral therapies being the most frequently used. The combination of antidepressant medication and cognitive-behavioral therapy has emerged as one of the most effective and beneficial treatment approaches for individuals with chronic mood disorders (Dunner 2001). As an example, in a study by Köhler et al. (2013) the addition of cognitive-behavioral therapy notably improved the outcome over standard procedure in the acute psychiatric treatment of inpatients with a unipolar depressive disorder. Studies have noted that the combination of pharmacotherapy and psychotherapy has provided greater psychosocial improvement (Hirschfeld et al. 2002), functioning, and quality of life (Kamenov et al. 2017). The combination of cognitive-behavioral therapy and pharmacotherapy also has a greater chance of a better outcome (lack of relapse or recurrence) than pharmacotherapy alone (Vittengl et al. 2007). Although there have been some systematic studies to date of the combination of medication with psychodynamic psychotherapies (Burnand et al. 2002; de Jonghe et al. 2001), it still remains difficult to determine which one is most effective for a particular patient. Furthermore, most current studies are trying to compare psychodynamic treatments with medication rather than assessing possible synergistic benefits of the combination of psychotherapy and pharmacotherapy (Roose 2001). In addition, some studies address functioning versus quality of life and use the terms interchangeably even though they are not identical (Kamenov et al. 2017; Lam et al. 2015), as *functioning* refers to performance in daily or social activities and *quality of life* refers to satisfaction with these activities and perception of health (IsHak et al. 2011). The Canadian Network for Mood and Anxiety Treatments, for example, highlighted the need for evidence-based interventions that demonstrate improvement in functioning, because patients have prioritized functional over symptomatic outcomes and determined the return to a normal level of functioning at work, home, or school as significant factors and aspects for remission in depression (Kamenov et al. 2017; Zimmerman et al. 2006).

As Frank et al. (2005) note in their very informative review on combining antidepressants and psychotherapy for depression, we need more information about the relative efficacy of pharmacotherapy and psychotherapy in combination versus each modality alone. Frank et al. point out that the majority of private practitioners, at least in the United States, see combination as the ideal treatment. The authors also note that in addition to more information about efficacy, we also need to know "how combination treatment is best practiced, i.e., what are the advantages and disadvantages to both treatments being provided by a single practitioner versus pharmacotherapist-psychotherapist treatment teams working in coordination versus completely independent practitioners providing pharmacotherapy and psychotherapy to the same individual" (Frank et al., p. 269). They also suggested that we need to know which model is most economical.

Gitlin and Miklowitz (2016) note that there are no data on the question of whether patients in integrated versus split/collaborative treatment differ in short- or long-term outcomes. Furthermore, there are very few studies that have adequately compared the cost of split/collaborative versus integrated treatment and then compared this to outcomes (Dewan 1999). In a 1995 claims data study from a national managed mental health care organization, the adjusted mean cost of outpatient services for depressed patients was significantly higher in a split/collaborative treatment group than in an integrated treatment group. This difference could have been related to the greater number of sessions, both of therapy and medication visits, in the split/collaborative treatment group, increasing the overall frequency of visits (Goldman et al. 1998).

Although this is all true, there still need to be guideposts for the training of residents. Psychiatry residents should be guided through the various issues to be considered in prescribing psychotropic medication and providing psychotherapy as part of integrated treatment.

Once a working diagnosis is developed, the resident must think through a series of issues related to medication and psychotherapy. In this chapter, we explore the various dimensions of the relationship between medication and psychotherapy to provide a practical framework for residents. Without much systematic data, we are left to use clinical experiences as a major basis for recommendations.

Sequence

There has historically been a dualism in psychiatry as shown by the Axis I–Axis II dichotomy, with a split regarding dynamic theories and medication. Many psychoanalysts, for example, view medication as an adjunct to the dynamic theory to be used only if the dynamic treatment is not sufficient. At the other end of the spectrum are primary care physicians or biologically oriented psychiatrists who use psychotropic medication and then make a referral to a mental health professional for psychotherapy if the patient is not improving with medication alone.

Furthermore, in DSM-IV and DSM-IV-TR, Axis III diagnoses were also critically important. Although DSM-5 does not use the multiaxial approach, it is still important to appreciate the impact of medical and surgical conditions and history, including medication. The resident needs to understand what medications the patient is currently taking, the patient's past and present medical history, the patient's family medical history, the patient's allergies, and any other symptoms that might be related to an underlying medical condition. If a patient has not been seen by his or her primary care physician or other physician for quite a while, it might be a good idea to suggest a checkup. If the patient has current and complicated medical problems, it might be a good idea for the psychiatry resident to receive permission to call the primary care physician to discuss the patient's current medical condition and to inquire as to whether the physician has any thoughts about the treatment plan for the current psychiatric problems.

The resident will want to know the patient's weight, height, and vital signs (including blood pressure) at the initiation of any type of treatment. These indices may be regularly checked by the clinic or ordered by the resident at the first visit and at intervals thereafter. The resident should also have access to any recent laboratory reports on the patient that might be helpful, such as blood sugar, liver enzymes, and thyroid function as well as an electrocardiogram.

The approach used in most of medicine is to try one treatment first and see if it works. Combinations of medications are prescribed, but medications usually are not started in combination; instead, they are sequenced. This is done so that the clinician can observe the effectiveness of one medication; see if there are any untoward effects, such as an allergic reaction; and then determine whether the medication is causing other side effects such as a sexual side effect, jitteriness, and so forth. In the past, when psychiatrists used to prescribe powerful antipsychotic medications with antidopaminergic and anticholinergic effects (e.g., thioridazine, chlorpromazine, haloperidol), there was a strong focus on treating the side effects early to keep the patient comfortable and to ensure adherence to the medication regimen. There was also the desire to make sure that these medications did not mask symptoms of tardive dyskinesia, which could become irreversible. The tradition was to start with one medication and then add others to help augment the benefits or reduce some of the negative side effects.

In much the same way, in integrated treatment the psychiatrist usually starts with one type of treatment, sees how it works, and then adds another treatment if necessary. It is valuable to document treatment carefully at each stage and to vary only one intervention at a time, so that the presence or absence of desired results can be tracked closely. In integrated treatment, depending on the nature and severity of the illness, the resident could start with either medication or psychotherapy and then add the other, or start with both medication and psychotherapy at the same time. Sequencing is a complex (Beitman et al. 2003), though effective, strategy (Guidi et al. 2011, 2016).

Diagnosis matters, because with patients who have depression or anxiety, providing medication first and dampening down symptoms might allow the patient to more fully participate in a form of psychotherapy later. Similarly, patients with a psychotic disorder may be suspicious, hallucinating, delusional, or manic and may need to be medicated first to feel more comfortable sitting and talking with a physician.

A good clinician will fully appreciate that symptoms and experiences of patients are seldom simple and straightforward. A suspicious, paranoid patient is not going to take medication prescribed by a clinician unless there is a good doctor–patient alliance. The patient needs to feel at least a little bit hopeful that the doctor means well and that the medicine is going to help make the patient feel better, rather than cause harm. The doctor–patient alliance is based on talk and the formation of a partnership between the doctor and patient. This talk could be part of supportive psychotherapy, interpersonal psychotherapy, or a type of cognitive-behavioral psychotherapy. Thus, one could argue that medication and psychotherapy are not truly sequenced because they are both integral components.

With that said, in determining a treatment plan the psychiatry resident should discuss with the patient all proven, effective types of treatment. Such types of treatment should at least be discussed, even if the clinician cannot personally provide the treatment. The patient should, nevertheless, be informed of all the options that are available, at a level commensurate with his or her educational and cognitive level.

Informed consent is the ethical and legal practice in which patients are engaged in a discussion about the nature of their condition and its likely progression without intervention and the different options for treatment. The anticipated benefits and risks associated with the different options, including nontreatment, should be explored, and every effort should be made to support the patient's voluntary decision making regarding his or her care. For many reasons, psychiatric conditions may sometimes interfere with patients' abilities to make sound and authentic decisions. To the extent possible, patients should be given the opportunity to make choices related to their care, even if additional safeguards (e.g., guardianship) become necessary to protect patient health, rights, and safety.

Toward these aims, in integrated care the patient should be provided with information about the kinds of psychotropic medication and psychotherapy the clinician is considering: whether one or the other or both should be used, and whether one should start before the other, and if not, why not. Patients arrive with expectations about what the psychiatrist will do: some are afraid that doctors are "pill pushers"; some have had good experiences with medications and want the doctor to give them pills to help take away painful symptoms; some view doctors as uncaring people who are too busy to really listen to patients and just want to write a prescription or order a consultation to send the patient off; and some view doctors as money-seeking practitioners who are just in it to get rich. Although many of these are negative constructs, most patients are very respectful and hopeful that the psychiatrist can help. Furthermore, with the present shortage of psychiatrists, patients have often had to wait a long time to see a doctor and may have more advanced symptoms because of the wait, which could add to the patient's frustration but also help in the building of a therapeutic alliance with the psychiatrist.

Starting With Medication

The diagnosis is critical to the resident's decision as to whether to prescribe medication in the beginning of treatment. It is important to determine how the patient feels about medication. If the patient is frightened, does not have the money to pay for medication, or has concomitant medical conditions for which more information is needed from the primary or specialty care physician, then holding off on prescribing early would be advisable. On the other hand, if the patient has a diagnosis amenable to medication (e.g., recurrent major depression) and has not been taking antidepressant medication since the last episode, it might be very reasonable to consider prescribing antidepressant medication in the very early stages of the treatment plan. The resident might consider providing antidepressant medication and discussing possible side effects, what to expect by taking the medication, and what might be added later (an augmenting agent or psychotherapy). In addition, there may be somatic problems that need to be treated sooner if the antidepressant does not address problems such as falling asleep, staying asleep, or daytime anxiety. The resident should understand ways the medication could potentially interfere with treatment, including possible interactions with other medications the patient is taking, and these should be evaluated.

If the patient continues with the antidepressant medication and starts feeling less sad and hopeless, he or she may begin to tell the clinician about stressors or triggers at the start of the depressive episode. If there are issues that relate to family members, psychotherapy might be most suitably administered as couples or family therapy; or with problems in organization or work relationships, cognitive-behavioral treatment might be most suitable. Psychiatrists often like to see the patient have fewer somatic problems and fewer acute problems before moving away from focusing on medication and concentrating more on problem solving.

Setting certainly plays an important part in sequencing. For example, if the first contact with the patient is in the emergency setting, medication might be provided first before psychotherapy because the symptoms presented are usually more acute and the follow-up care will be provided by another physician. Similarly, in the inpatient setting, where stays are quite short, medication might be provided before a course of psychotherapy.

However, in the outpatient setting, where the resident will be providing integrated treatment, the diagnosis, the patient's expectations, and the acuity of symptoms are probably the most significant factors in determining whether medication will be provided at the outset.

Even though medication might be warranted, another issue for the resident to consider is whether it might be more judicious to simply wait and see. What this means is that the patient might look different or present differently after a few sessions. What seems like anxiety early on might settle down very quickly as the patient gets to know the resident, and other symptoms or problems might emerge that may be more amenable to other types of treatment. What seems like an adjustment disorder with depressed mood may turn out to be an adjustment disorder that may resolve after several psychotherapy sessions, or it may turn out to be major depression, for which medication is warranted.

Sometimes the clinician is unsure of the working diagnosis, and in such cases, it might be prudent to wait before prescribing medication. Once medication has been started, it is harder to pull back or stop it. If a patient develops an untoward side effect, it might be more difficult to persuade the patient to try a higher dosage of the medication or even a different class of drug. It may be also useful to discuss the overall efficacy versus individual efficacy with the patient at the outset of treatment and emphasize that the success of treatment is "never guaranteed," that other medications may need to be tried if the first one does not work, and that the prescribing physician "will be trying his or her best."

Starting With Psychotherapy

If a form of psychotherapy is indicated, it is usually helpful to begin with education about the patient's diagnosis, what kinds of treatment are indicated and what type of psychotherapy is recommended. Patients like to know how long the treatment will last, what they should expect, whether they will be somehow different after it is complete, and what happens if the treatment is not successful. Patients may come in with a personal experience or experience of family members regarding psychotherapy. It is helpful for the clinician to know about this experience and to put the recommended form of therapy in context with what the patient may already know.

What is difficult for psychiatry residents is that although they need to educate and inform patients, they themselves may not yet have the clinical experience or background to fully answer all the questions. Furthermore, the resident might not have completed a particular form of psychotherapy with a patient with a similar problem and may be anxious about whether or not he or she can deliver the proper type of care. A supervisor will often help the resident through the first couple of cases with a particular type of psychotherapy, and even though the patient might be aware of this level of supervision, the resident might be in the unenviable position of feeling very alone in the provision of care.

It is therefore to be expected if the resident does not feel confident that a form of psychotherapy is definitely going to work or be successful. It is a difficult position to be in for the resident and for the patient, but just recognizing that this is the situation may help the resident to request more supervision and may allow for the patient to work more closely in partnership with the resident. Patients who choose teaching hospitals usually realize that the opportunity to work with bright, energetic trainees is a plus, even if they are not as seasoned and experienced as others in practice. The financial benefit of seeing a trainee might be a determining factor, or the availability and proximity of the institution may be the limiting issues.

There are, of course, situations for the provision of psychotherapy and medication in which consultation or referral is warranted because the patient is not doing well, the resident realizes that he or she cannot provide the needed care, or a combination of both. These decisions should be discussed with the supervisor, and the emphasis should always be in favor of providing what is best for the patient. Weighing these issues and making sure that the resident is not referring based on his or her own novice anxiety is very complex and is part of the training process.

When psychotherapy is begun initially, the focus is usually on dynamic issues and principles. Cognitive-behavioral therapy is a very important type of treatment for a wide range of disorders, including anxiety, depression, and substance abuse. When a patient's symptoms emerge that might be treated with medication, it is up to the resident to determine the risks and benefits of treating those symptoms with medication versus allowing the dynamic process to evolve. Again, the diagnosis is critical, and the working diagnosis should constantly be revisited. What started out as mild depression could over time develop into moderate or severe major depression that needs to be treated with medication. Continuing a form of psychotherapy without raising the possibility of using antidepressants might be quite risky. Similarly, a patient with a history of posttraumatic stress disorder might be presenting with mild symptoms of mood problems, yet with psychotherapy, there could be a reviewing of the initial trauma that could result in disequilibrium in anxiety and mood symptoms. Reassessment might lead to the conclusion that there needs to be an addition of medication to the psychotherapy regimen.

Competency

Psychiatry residents must be able to demonstrate the ability to form a working therapeutic alliance at the beginning of treatment.

Competency

Psychiatry residents must be able to demonstrate the ability to appreciate the issues that involve sequencing of medication (and/or other medical treatments) and psychotherapy.

Maintenance

It is difficult for most people to maintain anything, from an optimum weight, to good grades, to high job performance. We all have to work at maintenance: our dentists need to send us reminders about getting regular checkups; our cars have lights in the dashboard that come on to tell us that service needs to be performed; and so on. Most of us get bored or tired of doing the same thing day in and day out. We get complacent about how things are going; we want to see what will happen if we stop doing something that we regularly do; we want to see if there are cheaper or easier ways to get the same result.

A critical phase of treatment begins when the patient has become stable on medication and psychotherapy. The resident might be quite pleased about how the patient is doing, and so might the patient. But taking pills every day, coming to see the resident regularly, and paying the pharmacy and the clinic when feeling relatively well might trigger the patient's desire to make changes. It is therefore an important time for the resident to realize that hard work must be done to make sure the patient's good health continues.

The maintenance phase, for example, is a good time to ask about sexual side effects. In the early phases of taking medication, when the patient might have been quite depressed and anxious, low libido or decreased interest in sex might not have been so important to the patient. As the patient begins to feel well and his or her significant other sees that he or she is doing better with life activities, sex might again become important. If the medication prescribed by the resident has the potential to alter the patient's sex drive, it is important to raise that issue. The patient might not want to bring this issue up to the resident because of the realization that the resident is going to urge the patient to keep taking the medication. The patient might therefore start cutting down the dosage to see what happens.

Another issue during the maintenance phase is paying for medication and treatment. Most patients have to at least make a copayment for these forms of treatment. It might become a burden for patients to be paying for these forms of treatment, so they might think about what could be cut from the regimen. Again, it is better for the resident to be proactive about bringing up these issues and to work in partnership with the patient on these matters.

Family problems that are sometimes pushed to the back burner during a patient's acute presentation of symptoms move forward during maintenance treatment. Marital problems, parent–child issues, or financial troubles may all resurface as the patient starts improving. Bringing other family members into sessions with the patient might be helpful. If the patient is receiving integrated treatment—medication and psychotherapy—the resident and the patient can determine when and how these collateral partners might be brought into the care.

Adherence

It is very difficult for anyone to strictly adhere to a treatment plan, especially taking medication. Most people do not like to take medication. How many people actually finish a full course of antibiotics? Often, as they begin to feel better, patients stop taking medication. The track record in primary care with antidepressants is bleak—after 6 months, most patients are not taking the full dosage of antidepressant medication that was initially prescribed by the primary care doctor.

Nonadherence with medication regimens can take many forms: not getting prescriptions filled; not taking medications as prescribed, either by taking too many pills or taking too few, or not taking them on the right schedule; taking medication while also using alcohol or other drugs; or stopping medication before the agreed-on time. Regarding psychotherapeutic treatment, nonadherence might mean not keeping appointments, canceling appointments at the last minute, arriving late, not paying for treatment, not bringing family members or other participants to treatment, or not completing homework assignments.

There are also other factors related to the patient's psychopathology that may affect nonadherence, including paranoia, suspiciousness, or psychosis; substance abuse; cognitive deficits, such as poor memory; severe depression that prompts psychomotor agitation and feelings of hopelessness or worthlessness; and pressure by family or friends to stop the medication for various reasons.

What can the psychiatry resident do to improve adherence with the prescribed treatment of medication and psychotherapy? Some suggestions are listed below.

- Most patients appreciate education about the form of treatment they are receiving. Although written materials are helpful, certain types of patients may find it more useful to receive information over the telephone or Internet. Fact sheets about the medication and psychotherapy are good adjuncts. Web sites, handouts, books, and pamphlets are often useful. Although it is true that some patients will be frightened by what they read and may feel that they are getting all the possible side effects that are listed, it is important that they receive the information and that they can then discuss it with the resident.
- Some patients will benefit from joining support groups or local chapters of organizations for those with the same or similar disorder. Therefore, it might be useful to refer patients to the National Alliance on Mental Illness (NAMI), the Depression and Bipolar Support Alliance (DBSA), Alcoholics Anonymous (AA), Narcotics Anonymous (NA), or Al-Anon.
- Bringing family members into certain sessions might be very useful. Asking the patient's partner—spouse, girlfriend, or boyfriend—about how best to help the patient adhere to treatment can be beneficial.
- It is important to continue to ask patients about side effects and the state of their general medical health. Patients will realize that the clinician is continually vigilant about their medications and wants to make sure that things are going well. When might be a good time to decrease the dosage or stop the medication is a good topic for conversation. Sometimes patients might think that the clinician wants them to take the medication indefinitely, when that might not be the case at all.
- Pharmaceutical companies do a lot of direct-to-consumer advertising. If there is a big media blitz about a specific medication, it might be useful to ask patients what they have heard and what they think about the medication. It might be appropriate to talk about why the new medication on the market is suitable or unsuitable for the patient.
- Many patients might want to take alternative or complementary medications or supplements obtained from health food stores or over the Internet. There

are various reasons why more and more people are looking to use such substances, but it is important to ask patients about such substances. A substance that a patient is using as a supplement might not have an adverse impact on the main form of psychiatric treatment, and there is a possibility that it will have an effect on or interact negatively with medication, so it is important to know what the patient is taking. It is always useful to discuss patient's reasons for looking for alternative or complementary medications and to warn about lack of efficacy, possible side effects, and interactions with prescribed medication whenever appropriate.

- To treat a concomitant medical problem, the patient's primary care physician or specialty physician might prescribe a new medication that interacts with the psychotropic medication. It is important to know this so that the dosage of the psychotropic medication (or the type of medication itself) can be changed before the patient stops taking it altogether, which could lead to an escalation in psychiatric symptoms.
- Packaging interventions—such as using daily or weekly dosing, liquid or sublingual preparations, blister packs, etc.—might be useful for some patients as a behavioral strategy.
- First impressions of the resident are important. If the resident physician seems competent and confident, the patient usually feels better about adhering to treatment.
- When patients drop out of psychodynamic treatment, reasons often include a weaker therapeutic alliance, less of a focus on the patient's affect, and less supportive and dynamic work during sessions (Piper et al. 1999).

Competency

Psychiatry residents must be able to demonstrate knowledge of the factors that are important for the individual patient to maintain and adhere to a treatment regimen.

Conclusion

It is very difficult to know, based on the literature, how best to sequence medication and psychotherapy for patients in general. Providing a good working diagnosis, developing a treatment plan that is agreed to by both the patient and the resident, and continuing to evaluate how the patient is doing are all ways to improve the course of care. Although beginning the treatment is hard, it is also difficult to manage the maintenance phase of integrated treatment—helping the patient to adhere to ongoing, regular use of medication and psychotherapy. It is important for psychiatry residents to ask patients how they are doing, even when they appear to be doing well, because that is the time when patients might try changes in treatment on their own, without speaking to the resident first. Listening for and attending to these difficult periods in treatment are crucial for the administration of optimal integrated care.

Residents may be anxious about their ability to provide optimal care for their patients. Schofield and Grant (2013) have done interesting work looking into improving psychotherapists' competence through clinical supervision, which is generally regarded as an essential professional activity and as a quality assurance mechanism. There are also many exciting and useful new models for training residents on psychopharmacology prescribing through participation in workshops (Kavanagh et al. 2017).

Residents should be aware of high-risk times for nonadherence to treatment, including, for example, the beginning of treatment before the doctor–patient relationship has been solidified and before the onset of a good therapeutic alliance. In addition, it often takes some time before a medication or psychotherapy begins to take effect or for the patient or family to see results. For those who are impatient or who are looking for reasons not to continue treatment, this could be viewed as a high-risk time. Later on, there may be fears of dependence or drug addiction, and transference issues between the patient and physician may be reasons for adherence problems. Transfer of care of psychotherapy patients is another particularly worrisome time because of feelings of closeness and attachment that can develop in long-term therapeutic relationships and complicated feelings on the part of patients and residents (Schen et al. 2013).

Psychotherapy and pharmacotherapy can be and frequently are adjunctive to one another. While medication is being started and the dosage adjusted, it is beneficial for the resident to help the patient stay engaged in pleasurable activities and functions that are or had been important parts of the patient's life. Medication clinics are very useful for many patients as a way to decrease stigma and provide education and support to the patient. Personalized attention from clinicians, nurses, and other mental health providers, either by telephone or e-mail, also appears to be very effective.

The resident should assume that adherence to psychotherapy and pharmacotherapy will be difficult for most patients. The patient's adherence to medical and mental health treatment should be reviewed. At each session, a significant amount of time should be spent on monitoring symptoms and checking on issues related to adherence, especially in the early stages of treatment. Problems that the patient is having with obtaining the medication, taking the medication, getting to appointments, doing homework assignments, and arranging for support from friends and family members should all be explored (Wetherell and Unützer 2003). Any problems with these issues should be identified proactively, and problem solving should be part of the treatment. More frequent contact—by telephone, office visits, or e-mail—should be explored. Bringing in family members or other support persons should be investigated. If the patient has cognitive deficits, having family members or others help would be an important factor for success.

It is imperative that the resident help to solve problems and find out about these issues without appearing threatening or angry about nonadherence. One goal of treatment is for the patient to be able to self-monitor and provide ways to improve adherence on his or her own, for both medication and psychotherapy. It is important for the patient to feel that any problems can be addressed and discussed with the resident to make the treatment as successful as possible.

References

Beitman BD, Blinder BJ, Thase ME, et al: Integrating Psychotherapy and Pharmacotherapy: Dissolving the Mind-Brain Barrier. New York, WW Norton, 2003

Burnand Y, Andreoli A, Kolatte E, et al: Psychodynamic psychotherapy and clomipramine in the treatment of major depression. Psychiatr Serv 53(5):585–590, 2002 11986508

de Jonghe F, Kool S, van Aalst G, et al: Combining psychotherapy and antidepressants in the treatment of depression. J Affect Disord 64(2–3):217–229, 2001 11313088

Dewan M: Are psychiatrists cost-effective? An analysis of integrated versus split treatment. Am J Psychiatry 156(2):324–326, 1999 9989575

Dunner DL: Acute and maintenance treatment of chronic depression. J Clin Psychiatry 62 (suppl 6):10–16, 2001 11310814

Frank E, Novick D, Kupfer DJ: Antidepressants and psychotherapy: a clinical research review. Dialogues Clin Neurosci 7(3):263–272, 2005 16156384

Gitlin MJ, Miklowitz DJ: Split treatment: recommendations for optimal use in the care of psychiatric patients. Ann Clin Psychiatry 28(2):132–137, 2016 27285393

Goldman W, McCulloch J, Cuffel B, et al: Outpatient utilization patterns of integrated and split psychotherapy and pharmacotherapy for depression. Psychiatr Serv 49(4): 477–482, 1998 9550237

Guidi J, Fava GA, Fava M, et al: Efficacy of the sequential integration of psychotherapy and pharmacotherapy in major depressive disorder: a preliminary meta-analysis. Psychol Med 41(2):321–331, 2011 20444307

Guidi J, Tomba E, Fava GA: The sequential integration of pharmacotherapy and psychotherapy in the treatment of major depressive disorder: a meta-analysis of the sequential model and a critical review of the literature. Am J Psychiatry 173(2):128–137, 2016 26481173

Hirschfeld RM, Dunner DL, Keitner G, et al: Does psychosocial functioning improve independent of depressive symptoms? A comparison of nefazodone, psychotherapy, and their combination. Biol Psychiatry 51(2):123–133, 2002 11822991

IsHak WW, Greenberg JM, Balayan K, et al: Quality of life: the ultimate outcome measure of interventions in major depressive disorder. Harv Rev Psychiatry 19(5):229–239, 2011 21916825

Kamenov K, Twomey C, Cabello M, et al: The efficacy of psychotherapy, pharmacotherapy and their combination on functioning and quality of life in depression: a meta-analysis. Psychol Med 47(3):414–425, 2017 27780478

Kavanagh EP, Cahill J, Arbuckle MR, et al: Psychopharmacology prescribing workshops: a novel method for teaching psychiatry residents how to talk to patients about medications. Acad Psychiatry February 13, 2017 [Epub ahead of print] 28194682

Köhler S, Hoffmann S, Unger T, et al: Effectiveness of cognitive-behavioural therapy plus pharmacotherapy in inpatient treatment of depressive disorders. Clin Psychol Psychother 20(2):97–106, 2013 22095701

Lam RW, Parikh SV, Michalak EE, et al: Canadian Network for Mood and Anxiety Treatments (CANMAT) consensus recommendations for functional outcomes in major depressive disorder. Ann Clin Psychiatry 27(2):142–149, 2015 25954941

Piper WE, Ogrodniczuk JS, Joyce AS, et al: Prediction of dropping out in time-limited, interpretive individual psychotherapy. Psychotherapy 36:114–122, 1999

Roose SP: Psychodynamic therapy and medication: can treatments in conflict be integrated? in Integrated Treatment of Psychiatric Disorders. Edited by Kay J (Review of Psychiatry series; Oldham JM and Riba MB, series eds). Washington, DC, American Psychiatric Publishing, 2001, pp 31–49

Schen CR, Raymond L, Notman M: Transfer of care of psychotherapy patients: implications for psychiatry training. Psychodyn Psychiatry 41(4):575–595, 2013 24283450

Schofield MJ, Grant J: Developing psychotherapists' competence through clinical supervision: protocol for a qualitative study of supervisory dyads. BMC Psychiatry 13(12), 2013 23298408

Vittengl JR, Clark LA, Dunn TW, et al: Reducing relapse and recurrence in unipolar depression: a comparative meta-analysis of cognitive-behavioral therapy's effects. J Consult Clin Psychol 75(3):475–488, 2007 17563164

Wetherell JL, Unützer J: Adherence to treatment for geriatric depression and anxiety. CNS Spectr 8 (12, suppl 3):48–59, 2003 14978463

Zimmerman M, McGlinchey JB, Posternak MA, et al: How should remission from depression be defined? The depressed patient's perspective. Am J Psychiatry 163(1):148–150, 2006 16390903

Selection of Medication, Psychotherapy, and Clinicians in Split/Collaborative Treatment

5

There are several different circumstances under which a resident might provide split/collaborative treatment for a patient. Some of the possible circumstances include the following:

1. The patient is seen by the resident for a psychiatric evaluation. In the course of the evaluation, the resident determines that it would be best for the patient to see another clinician (usually a social worker or psychologist) for psychotherapy, while the resident continues to see the patient for medication and medical issues related to the treatment.
2. The patient is seen by the resident for a psychiatric evaluation. In the course of the evaluation, the patient tells the resident that he or she is already seeing a therapist and was referred for medication. If the resident feels that medication is warranted, then the resident would be the provider of the psychotropic medication and other pertinent medical issues only.

3. The patient is already being seen by a therapist. A primary care physician or other physician has been treating the patient with psychotropic medication, but the patient is not improving, so the physician sends the patient to the clinic for more expert evaluation and treatment by the resident.

4. The patient is seeing a resident for integrated treatment—psychotherapy and medication—but the psychotherapy part of the care will end (e.g., both the patient and resident agree that psychotherapy is no longer needed, insurance benefits changed, the patient can no longer afford therapy, the patient decides that he or she does not want psychotherapy), so the resident continues to see the patient for medication and medical management.

In all the situations outlined above, there are particular decisions that the resident and supervisor must make in determining the proper care for the patient. What is the resident able and competent to provide? What should be the timing and sequencing of medication and psychotherapy? Whom should the resident refer the patient to, based on the need for a certain type of psychotherapy?

As noted in other chapters of this book and by several authors (e.g., Busch and Sandberg 2012), the split/collaborative treatment arrangement could be a source of conflict between the two care providers and the patient. Busch and Sandberg (2012, p. 174) note that "competitive and professional tensions, as well as different theoretical models, can generate problems in treatment management. Patients may idealize and devaluate one or the other of the clinicians, or act out in ways that may be difficult to address. A triadic therapeutic alliance and communication about problems have been recommended as ways of identifying and addressing problems."

Another related complicating issue that should be addressed from the outset of the split/collaborative arrangement is lack of communication between care providers (e.g., Gitlin and Miklowitz 2016; Hansen-Grant and Riba 1995). Routine contact between psychopharmacologist and therapist is much less frequent than expected (Gitlin and Miklowitz 2016). Kahn (1991) discussed practical techniques in split/collaborative treatment, suggesting several issues that should be discussed during the initial conversation between psychopharmacologist and therapist.

Communication should be established from the very beginning of the split/collaborative treatment and should include issues such as the treatment contract, clarification of each clinician's responsibilities, agreement on regular contact between clinicians, and possible collaborative work on the patient treatment plan (Hansen-Grant and Riba 1995). If the resident has referred the patient to another clinician for psychotherapy, the resident should explain to the patient and to the psychotherapist what medication(s) will be prescribed, what the expected outcome is, what possible major side effects could occur, and when and how to contact the prescriber in case of side effects. As Gitlin and Miklowitz (2016) suggest, communication should occur at important treatment junctures, such as major change in diagnosis (e.g., unipolar depression to bipolar disorder), major change in symptomatology (e.g., substance abuse, psychosis), and new-onset or marked exacerbation of suicidal ideation or risk. (Here, Gitlin and Miklowitz suggest that the therapist who is seeing the patient more frequently begin distributing a weekly supply of medication to the patient to mitigate the risk of overdose.)

The issues and tasks noted above are some of the most difficult for even seasoned clinicians. The resident must often make these assessments in a single evaluation while also trying to formulate a diagnosis and a treatment plan, assess strengths and weaknesses of the treatment plan and obstacles to its implementation, and ascertain access to care.

In this chapter, we highlight some of the specific issues that the resident needs to consider in the various scenarios described above, realizing that these situations are very fluid and can easily shift based on a wide variety of factors. This process is very complex and difficult, particularly because it is triangulated: it involves the patient, the resident, and another clinician who will be providing the primary treatment.

Scenario A: Referral to a Psychotherapist

In this scenario, the resident makes a decision, based on the evaluation, to refer the patient to another clinician for psychotherapy while continuing to see the patient for medication. What are the factors that would lead the resident to this recommendation?

The patient's history is quite important. The patient might tell the resident that he or she has had this type of split/collaborative treatment in the past and has done well with it. The resident might want to ask why the patient did not go back to the former care providers. It could be that the patient moved, that the previous care providers are no longer available, that it is inconvenient for the patient to seek treatment with the previous providers, or that the patient has a different type of insurance plan not covering the original care providers. It is important to clarify the reasons why the patient is seeking new clinicians.

The resident might feel that the patient would benefit from being seen frequently, but the resident's schedule might not allow for such frequency. For example, the patient may have a diagnosis of major depression and mild, recurrent, and multiple stressors, including a new job, that would require support and help from a clinician. The resident might determine that a course of medication would be useful and that supportive therapy might also be an important addition.

Another factor to consider is whether the patient would benefit from seeing a therapist for at least 2 years. If the resident is about to graduate or switch to another clinical post, it might be in the patient's best interest to be seen by someone who can provide more long-term care.

The patient might be unsure if he or she wants psychotherapy or is willing to make a commitment to be seen regularly for such treatment. In this situation, the resident might want to make sure that the medication is prescribed before making the recommendation for another therapist to see the patient. Or the patient might live a distance from the university or hospital and might be willing to come in for the medical care but might not be so sure regarding the psychotherapy.

Another factor could be a resident's real or perceived lack of expertise in a certain psychotherapy. For instance, a beginning resident might not feel comfortable providing psychodynamic psychotherapy for a complex case of depression when it is recommended by the supervisor to be added to medication. (There are studies demonstrating the efficacy of psychodynamic psychotherapy and medication in the treatment of major depression; see, e.g., Burnand et al. 2002.)

Competency

Psychiatry residents must be able to determine under what conditions split/collaborative treatment would be most appropriate for a patient and must be able to convey these issues to the patient.

Scenario B: Referral to the Resident

In this scenario, the patient has a strong bond with a therapist who has referred the patient to the resident for medication. It is important at this point to obtain a separate explanation from the therapist of the reason for the referral. The patient might have a perception that medication is needed. The therapist may feel that the treatment has reached an impasse, that the patient is not doing well, and that medication may be a possible solution. It is critically important for the resident to have a conversation with the referring therapist, preferably before evaluating the patient, so that the nature of the referral is made clear and the expectations of the therapist are understood.

The resident ideally should also understand what the patient is expecting from the evaluation. Is there an expectation that a pill will be prescribed? If there is no such expectation, what would that mean? The resident should perform a complete psychiatric evaluation without making any assumptions about the diagnosis, history, or treatment. This evaluation should be conducted as if it were a de novo evaluation, even if there has been a discussion with the referring therapist. The resident must hear the story from the patient, including all the components of a good evaluation: present illness, past psychiatric and medical history, family history, social history, review of systems, mental status, formulation, and so on.

The resident needs to understand the expectations of the patient, the referring therapist, and anyone else—family members, friends of the patient—regarding why the patient is being seen for a psychiatric evaluation. It may be that the resident needs to speak with the patient's family doctor or other medical specialist and obtain laboratory studies, recent psychiatric or medical inpatient records, or other information before determining a treatment plan and course of action. It is especially important to explore the patient's response to previous medications and side effects of previous treatments, if any. The resident might need to speak to the referring therapist about the diagnosis and treatment plan before deciding on a course of action, especially when there needs to be a decision about the use of benefits and sessions. The resident must also be able to refuse to provide pharmacotherapy if he or she feels that it is not indicated and must be able to convey this tactfully to the patient and to the referring therapist. This all should be explained to the patient (and possibly to family members) in a plain, understandable way.

In certain situations, the resident might determine that it would be more helpful to take over both the psychotherapy and medication for a period of time. The patient could then go back to the referring therapist when things are clarified and more stable. This kind of decision would have to be made carefully, with considerable attention being given to transference and countertransference issues for the patient and the referring therapist. The resident should also be certain about the reasons for this type of decision.

Competency

Psychiatry residents should be able to demonstrate the ability to determine their role in a split/collaborative treatment arrangement and to obtain the appropriate information from the patient, medical records, the referring therapist, other medical clinicians, family members, and other sources.

Scenario C: Referral of a Patient in Poor Condition

In this scenario, the patient has already been treated psychopharmacologically by another physician and is not doing well. Therefore, certain expectations have developed in the patient (and perhaps in the referring physician and therapist) about what the resident will be able to accomplish. At the beginning, it is important for the resident to talk with the referring physician and the therapist to better understand what has been tried pharmacologically, what type of psychotherapy has been provided, the sequence of medication and psychotherapy given, any improvement in symptoms, and other medical problems and medications. Written documentation from the referring physician, including medication logs (including dosages, symptoms, and refills), should be obtained. This will help the resident to review how long a medication trial lasted, whether the patient adhered to the trial regimen, how often medications were changed or combined, how often the patient was seen, and whether medication was monitored with visits or telephone calls.

It is also important for the resident to review all the medications with the patient, once again going over symptom changes, what made things worse or better, and any other factors that might have had an impact on the patient's use of the medication. Illustrating the course of treatment, medications used, side effects, and so forth in a graph might also be useful. Sometimes, it is also helpful, with the patient's consent, to bring a family member in for part of a session to go over his or her assessment of the patient's symptoms when taking medications. The family member will often have a different perception of the various issues surrounding medications. This also provides the resident with an opportunity to hear what other family members think of psychotropic medication and how they feel it affects the patient.

It might take some time to get all the information from the referring doctor, the therapist, the patient, and the family member, but the resident should not feel compelled to prescribe at the first or even second session. In this scenario, the patient has not had as good a recovery as the patient, the family, the doctor, or the therapist expected, so it is important to be as careful and as thoughtful as possible.

An important question that needs to be asked by the resident is whether the diagnosis that the referring doctor and therapist are using as the basis for medication is the correct diagnosis. Often, on closer review, the working diagnosis must be changed. The patient could have a substance use problem that was not previously uncovered. The patient could have an underlying personality disorder that was not previously understood, affecting the primary diagnosis and the outcome of treatment (Busch and Sandberg 2012; Colli et al. 2014). The patient may have developed a new medical condition (e.g., diabetes, cancer, hypothyroidism) that is affecting the outcome of treatment, or the patient may have added a new medication, over-the-counter supplement, or alternative medication that is negatively affecting his or her presentation of psychiatric symptoms. There could be new stressors, new pressures, a new relationship, or financial difficulties that are clearly germane to the current symptoms that the patient has not brought to the attention of the referring doctor or therapist.

Competency

Psychiatry residents should develop the ability to potentially reformulate a case.

Scenario D: Ending Psychotherapy

In this scenario, a significant change is made in the relationship between the resident and the patient. The resident will discontinue psychotherapy for the patient while continuing to provide medication and medical care. It is very important that this change take place with careful planning and agreement between the patient and the resident (and the resident's supervisor), because such a change is usually permanent.

The reason for the change and who is initiating the change should be clarified. For example, if the reason for ending the psychotherapy component of care is related to the patient's finances, the patient should admit this to the resident, and the possibility of restarting psychotherapy if the financial situation improves should be kept open. In this situation, it is important for the patient to understand that psychotherapy cannot be merged into the medication sessions with the hope of accomplishing the same goals. This could be disappointing for the patient, who might feel hurt when sessions become shorter and when the usual issues are not discussed and are not allowed to develop. Both the patient and the resident may feel frustrated and angry about this situation and may not understand where these feelings are coming from. As noted by Mintz (2005) and Schen et al. (2013), the patient's reaction to the loss of the psychotherapy relationship may go unnoticed by the resident, who may feel that the continuity of the relationship overrides the loss of psychotherapy.

If the patient is initiating the change in care, then the reasons should be carefully reviewed and understood. Does the patient feel that his or her problems are not improving and that the resident cannot help? Is the patient no longer able or willing to put the same effort into the treatment? Is the patient concerned that the resident will be leaving soon (e.g., graduating) and attempting to avoid putting more into the relationship? Is the patient embarrassed about certain aspects of the psychotherapy? Does the patient no longer trust the resident for some reason? Did something happen or was something said in a session that bothered the patient? Is the patient's improved self-understanding causing changes at home and instability in the family? It is important to understand and discuss all of these issues in order to give both the resident and the patient the opportunity to address them. Setting up a special supervision session may be helpful in such cases.

The resident and the patient need to discuss what will happen if the patient starts to decompensate or deteriorate and the resident feels that psychotherapy needs to be resumed. It is important for this discussion to occur before the psychotherapy is terminated to put a plan in place for such a situation.

It is also important to discuss the consideration that although medication may seem to have taken care of all the patient's problems, it might not have been as successful without the psychotherapy provided by the resident. Sometimes patients impart certain causes and effects to treatments that may be justified and valid, but it is often impossible to know for sure what was proximate to a successful outcome. Medications can become overvalued and idealized, and when psychotherapy is taken away it sometimes becomes clear that the medication was not solely responsible for the remedy. There needs to be a form of psychoeducation about the role of psychotherapy and pharmacotherapy, which may run counter to the patient's belief system.

Competency

Psychiatry residents need to demonstrate how best to terminate psychotherapy when both psychotherapy and pharmacotherapy are provided.

There are a few issues related to resident clinics specifically. One issue is the tendency to change medication (or, more frequently, a combination of medications) at the beginning of the outpatient psychiatry rotation, especially in chronic patients who seem to be only partially improved or not functioning well. Residents may spend the entire year trying to find the "right" medication or combination of medications, only to find out that the original medication or combination was "it." This could create a lot of negative transference and lead to conflict with the patient's therapist, who may be more familiar with the case.

Another issue specific to resident clinics involves repeated transfers. Schen et al. (2013, p. 580) recommend that "patients who have been repeatedly transferred require periodic reassessment in order to avoid becoming chronic transfer patients and acquiring a kind of second-class status…these patients, rather than developing an institutional transference, have adapted by detaching from the loss of multiple individuals. Their lack of response can make residents feel inadequate…" In these situations, communication and working together with the patient's therapist may be of invaluable help.

Conclusion

For the psychiatry resident, participating in a split/collaborative treatment arrangement is complex and difficult. Not only does the resident have to worry about the patient, but the resident also has to consider other clinicians—both what they are doing and thinking and the patient's past and present relationship with them. The resident must glean much more information and history from all parties involved. This requires thoroughness, a sense of direction, and an ability to demonstrate patience. The resident is asked to be an expert, to help a patient recover, and to develop a deeper understanding and appreciation of the patient without making current coproviders and previous providers appear inadequate or unable to solve the problem. A delicate balance is required for the resident; even the most experienced clinicians have difficulty walking this tightrope. The resident should master competencies related to the variable scenarios that are presented. The resident ideally will be able to take a longer view of the situation and not be too quick to pick up a prescription pad. Supervision is key to the successful treatment of patients in a split/collaborative treatment arrangement, but the resident often has many such patients in this kind of care. Nevertheless, it is critical that the resident seek out good supervision, especially for more complex and difficult cases.

References

Burnand Y, Andreoli A, Kolatte E, et al: Psychodynamic psychotherapy and clomipramine in the treatment of major depression. Psychiatr Serv 53(5):585–590, 2002 11986508

Busch FN, Sandberg LS: Combined treatment of depression. Psychiatr Clin North Am 35(1):165–179, 2012 22370497

Colli A, Tanzilli A, Dimaggio G, et al: Patient personality and therapist response: an empirical investigation. Am J Psychiatry 171(1):102–108, 2014 24077643

Gitlin MJ, Miklowitz DJ: Split treatment: recommendations for optimal use in the care of psychiatric patients. Ann Clin Psychiatry 28(2):132–137, 2016 27285393

Hansen-Grant S, Riba MB: Contact between psychotherapists and psychiatric residents who provide medication backup. Psychiatr Serv 46(8):774–777, 1995 7583476

Kahn DA: Medication consultation and split treatment during psychotherapy. J Am Acad Psychoanal 19(1):84–98, 1991 1676395

Mintz DL: Teaching the prescriber's role: the psychology of psychopharmacology. Acad Psychiatry 29(2):187–194, 2005 15937266

Schen CR, Raymond L, Notman M: Transfer of care of psychotherapy patients: implications for psychiatry training. Psychodyn Psychiatry 41(4):575–595, 2013 24283450

Evaluation and Opening in Split/Collaborative Treatment

6

In this chapter, we review the initial evaluation and opening of the treatment process of pharmacotherapy by a resident either 1) with a new patient who was referred by a nonmedical therapist or primary care physician for pharmacotherapy *while* the patient remains in therapy with the nonmedical therapist, or 2) with a new patient whom the resident evaluates and then decides that psychotherapy will be provided by another clinician for various reasons (e.g., time constraints; economic reasons [e.g., the third-party payer does not reimburse for psychotherapy provided by a psychiatrist]; lack of expertise in a specific area or with a specific population; geographic considerations). We address the initial evaluation and related competencies in each of these situations. There are of course many other combinations and permutations, but we believe these to be two of the major types of situations that should be understood by residents.

This chapter is similar to Chapter 3, "Evaluation and Opening in Integrated Treatment," because the initial evaluations in integrated treatment and split/ collaborative treatment bear many similarities. There are, however, issues specific to split/collaborative treatment that are important to point out and address. There has been some work done on the communication patterns between clinicians who are engaged in split/collaborative therapy. In one study by Kalman et al. (2012), split/collaborative therapy was common, but adequate communication between professionals did not take place. Hansen-Grant and Riba (1995), in a chart review study, found similar communication problems.

Our view is that all care should be collaborative and respectful and that if the psychiatrist or other physician is not collaborating or communicating with the nonmedical therapist, this is not optimal split/collaborative treatment.

Initial Evaluation

As we noted in Chapter 3 for integrated treatment, the initial evaluation of any patient starts during the first contact with the patient, whether this occurs over the telephone with a managed care intermediary, with a nurse who is collecting information, with a receptionist, or with someone else. The patient begins to form an opinion of the clinician even before the first visit based on this initial contact.

The initial evaluation is mainly about collecting data that the psychiatrist considers pertinent for making a diagnosis and deciding on a treatment plan—in this case, usually pharmacotherapy. Again, it should not be forgotten that the initial evaluation is also about forming the therapeutic alliance with the patient.

The referral for pharmacotherapy could be initiated by a nonmedical therapist who is well known to the evaluating resident and who will closely work with the psychiatrist for truly collaborative treatment. This situation occurs frequently in residency training programs in which residents get referrals for pharmacotherapy from nonmedical therapist faculty members, staff members, or trainees (e.g., psychologists, social workers, psychology interns).

However, the request for the initial evaluation and subsequent pharmacotherapy may be initiated by a nonmedical therapist not known to the resident or as a self-referral by the patient. We would like to emphasize that no matter who the referral source is and under what circumstances the referral was made, the initial evaluation should be the same: very thorough and detailed. Nothing should be left unexplored just because this information has already been obtained by the referral source and provided to the evaluating resident. Accepting the interpretation of others could be misleading, and information from the referral source should be checked with the patient. Reinterpretation of clinical data by using newly collected information can be essential to pharmacotherapy planning.

We have frequently seen a written referral for pharmacotherapy with a very specific request—for example, "Please evaluate patient for initiation of treatment with a selective serotonin reuptake inhibitor." Such requests should be viewed with caution and carefully evaluated. A request from a nonmedical therapist should be discussed with the patient, and the resident should clarify whether the patient understands and agrees with the request. It should also be made clear that the request will not be automatically honored. The resident should make sure the patient understands that the decision to initiate pharmacotherapy and the selection of the specific pharmacotherapy will be based on the initial evaluation and on possible laboratory and other evaluations. The resident should also explain to the patient that the decision about pharmacotherapy will be made in the best interests of the patient, based on the resident's best expertise and professional opinion. Thus, the resident's task may include overcoming some resistance and preconceived ideas about which pharmacotherapeutic agent should be chosen and what pharmacotherapy should be like. (For example, a nonmedical therapist may suggest to the patient that all of his or her patients have been doing well with some particular medication, whereas the patient's symptomatology may require medication with a different efficacy or tolerance profile.) The initial evaluation also presents a good opportunity to determine whether the patient has any negative thoughts about being treated by a resident and to review what type of supervision the resident will be given regarding the patient's care.

It should be made clear to the patient and to the referring therapist that the first session (or first few sessions) will be devoted to an evaluation and that only after its completion will any decision about pharmacotherapy be made. Also, to avoid further misconceptions and false expectations, the resident should inform the patient or the therapist of the length of the initial evaluation, because some outside therapists may tell patients that the resident will spend just a few minutes with them. Bender and Messner (2003) suggest that the first session be framed as a consultation and evaluation; this allows the patient and the psychiatrist to evaluate whether they are a good match and whether they feel comfortable working with each other. Framing the first contact as a consultation is much easier in an outpatient setting.

Conceptualizing the initial evaluation as a consultation may also better reflect the reality of the initial evaluation. Nonmedical therapists mostly refer patients for initiation of pharmacotherapy, but the foremost question of the referral is consultative: "Is pharmacotherapy indicated, and if it is indicated, would you initiate and prescribe?" The question of whether pharmacotherapy is indicated should always be carefully pondered. Nonmedical therapists may at times and for various reasons get stalled in therapy and may refer the patient for pharmacotherapy as a last resort, but pharmacotherapy may not necessarily be the best solution. Countertransference may play a major role in the therapist's request for pharmacological consultation. Therefore, if after a careful initial evaluation the resident concludes that pharmacotherapy is not indicated, the resident should resist any pressure from the patient or therapist and should refuse to initiate pharmacotherapy. Having a discussion with the nonmedical therapist and suggesting a different therapeutic approach or even a different psychotherapy might be more appropriate.

Competency

Psychiatry residents must be able to understand the various dynamic and biological reasons for the request for a psychopharmacological consultation and must be able to obtain the appropriate information to make an informed decision about the diagnosis and treatment plan.

The initial step in the evaluation in both situations—either with a patient who was referred to the resident or with a patient who is seen de novo and will be referred for psychotherapy to a nonmedical therapist—is to establish an accurate diagnosis. It is important to reemphasize, however, that the diagnosis does not provide much information about the patient or the patient's needs in treatment planning. Factors such as symptoms, cooperation or resistance, family history, medical history, support system, previous treatment experience, previous medications, and value and belief system should be explored in the first session (or sessions) to help inform the decision about treatment. Much of this information should be included in the referral note or initial evaluation by the nonmedical therapist when the patient is referred for an evaluation by a nonmedical therapist or by a primary care provider. Nevertheless, we emphasize that this information needs to be checked and probed again.

First Contact: Technical and Introductory Remarks

The patient may arrive with various preconceived ideas and expectations. For example, the patient may have been referred to the resident after a more or less unsuccessful course of therapy, or the patient may have some negative transference feelings that have built up during the course of therapy and he or she may believe that physicians are all cold and uninterested or "just pushing pills."

As noted in Chapter 3, in this era of increased concerns about confidentiality, the resident needs to make sure that the patient's identity is protected. Therefore, calling the patient by last name in the waiting area might be problematic because it reveals the patient's identity, but calling the patient by first name may not fare well with older patients. Experts (e.g., Bender and Messner 2003) advise psychiatrists to simply identify the patient who is waiting and then invite the patient to follow or come in.

For the psychiatry resident, one of the most difficult aspects of split/collaborative treatment is figuring out who is really responsible for the patient's care. The answer, however, is clear: the physician is ultimately responsible, professionally and in the eyes of the law. Nevertheless, confusion can arise when the patient has had a long-standing relationship with a therapist and is coming to see the resident specifically for medication. The resident will want to evaluate the patient, obtain a full history, and make an assessment, but the patient might not understand why the resident requires so much information. The patient may wonder why the resident cannot obtain this information from the medical record or from the therapist. The patient might not understand why he or she has to provide all this information again.

In the case of an evaluation in a split/collaborative treatment arrangement, especially when the patient is referred for the evaluation by a therapist, some of the central questions that the patient and the resident need to address are as follows:

- Why is this evaluation being requested now?
- What are the patient's expectations?
- What are the referring therapist's expectations?
- What is the expected outcome of this evaluation?
- What are the goals of this session?
- What is the patient's level of understanding?
- Does the resident have enough information to do a complete evaluation at this session? Will there need to be one or more follow-up sessions to complete the evaluation?
- What is the level of confidentiality between the patient and the resident? How much will the resident discuss with the referring therapist? What are the lines of communication between the psychiatrist and the therapist, and how frequently will they be used? It is important for the resident to note that confidentiality does not apply here and that the Health Insurance Portability and Accountability Act (HIPAA) rules are frequently misinterpreted.
- What is the patient's diagnosis according to the resident? Is this diagnosis different than the diagnosis provided by the referring therapist?
- Which mental health professional should be contacted for which problems? The patient should be instructed to contact the psychiatrist regarding any issues related to medication and also for other clinical issues, such as feeling worse or suicidal.

The resident ideally should think about these complicated issues even before seeing the patient.

Competency

Psychiatry residents should be able to determine the multiple issues that need to be addressed in the initial evaluation of a patient being referred by an outside therapist or physician or as a self-referral.

As noted in Chapter 3, the resident should be observant of the patient's behavior during the initial period of evaluation. The resident should also inform the patient that confidential notes will be taken if this is the case. As MacKinnon and Yudofsky (1991, p. 10) note, some patients may be resentful if the resident takes *no* notes during the interview because it would make them feel that the resident was uninterested, whereas other patients cannot tolerate note taking because they feel that it distracts the psychiatrist's attention from them.

Many psychiatrists start the initial evaluation by obtaining basic patient data such as age, marital status, and employment, while others advocate beginning the session with an open-ended question. When the patient has been referred by a nonmedical therapist, the resident could begin the session with the question, "What is your understanding of why you have been sent to see me?" A further explanatory comment might also be helpful, such as "I understand that you were referred to me by your therapist, but what I am interested in is why you originally went to see your therapist and what has happened since then." The patient should be left to answer this question without interruption if possible.

The resident and the residency training director should make sure that the clinic provides at least 1 hour to see a new patient for a psychiatric evaluation. Some clinics provide only 30 minutes, based on the assumption that the referring clinician has already performed an evaluation. Thirty minutes is not adequate for any initial evaluation even for an experienced clinician; it is certainly not enough time for a resident at any stage of training. The resident must gather a large amount of information in the evaluation and, most importantly, form a therapeutic alliance with the patient, which is more difficult to achieve when the patient already has an alliance with another clinician or therapist. In addition, the resident and patient should discuss prescribed medication and documentation, which takes a significant amount of time. In the event that a resident must transition out of service for a patient in a split/collaborative treatment arrangement, the incoming resident who will take over the case should ideally see the patient for 1 hour for a new evaluation. The patient should ideally not be charged for this new evaluation; it should be billed as a follow-up. This provides the resident with the opportunity to appropriately treat and learn about the patient but does not encumber the patient with an extra expense due to the nature of the teaching service. The resident ideally should not be asked to do too many of these initial evaluations, as they are complicated and take so much time (both in the session and outside the session), much of which is not billable.

With these types of "handoffs" much of the first session might be about the patient's loss. As Schen et al. (2013) point out, the patient may feel rejected or abandoned by the loss of the previous resident. "Depending on the length and expectations of treatment, the depth of the therapeutic relationship, and the patient's character structure and history of attachments, patients respond to and manage the transfer with a wide range of emotional responses" (Schen et al. 2013,

p. 576). Although the resident may be focused on getting a full evaluation, the patient may need help to deal with this loss.

Furthermore, it is important for the resident to have an opportunity to receive supervision after seeing the patient. Many university clinics have an attending psychiatrist sit in on the evaluation session for key portions of the case. However, this may not provide adequate time for the resident to digest the information, think about the formulation and treatment plan, and provide psychoeducation to the patient with the supervisor's guidance. It may be necessary either to ask the patient to leave the office for a few minutes or to have the resident and supervisor leave the office for a few minutes to discuss the diagnosis and treatment plan together. However, such an arrangement may trigger transferential feelings and prompt the patient to wonder who is in charge. We have had good experience with residents briefly discussing the case with the supervisor at the end of the evaluation in the supervisor's office (not in the hallway) and later discussing the case in more detail in a case conference with the supervisor and, ideally, with another clinical or psychotherapy supervisor present. Schofield and Grant (2013) have outlined a qualitative study to help improve psychotherapists' competence through clinical supervision.

Although time with the patient may be viewed as a luxury, it is something that is very necessary. The patient should be scheduled for a follow-up to determine 1) whether the patient appears the same or different, 2) whether the symptoms with which the patient presents are the same or have changed, and 3) whether the patient will return for the follow-up appointment. The resident should not settle on a patient's formulation, diagnosis, and treatment plan prematurely. Providing the wrong medication or making the wrong diagnostic assessment can set the patient back for a long time and can have a negative impact on the therapeutic alliance between the patient and the resident (and future clinicians). Potentially, the wrong medication could cause morbidity or even death in the patient. If a prescription is provided at the first session and the patient does not return for follow-up, this could add to potential liability and other problems for the resident and the clinic. This is particularly problematic with certain high-risk patients, such as suicidal patients or patients with character pathology (McNary 2016).

Competency

Psychiatry residents must be able to balance the number of patients in split/collaborative treatment with the complex and time-consuming nature of evaluating and treating such patients.

One of the ways to address the points outlined above is to educate the patient about why it is so complicated to conduct an evaluation. The resident should explain that it is not because the patient is very sick or difficult, which is what the patient might be worried about, but rather because it will take a while to do a thorough job. Most patients can appreciate that it is complicated to prescribe medication, check side effects and medication interactions, consider age issues, and evaluate the effects of other medical problems. Most patients will agree that hastily prescribing a medication to see if it works is not in the best interest of either the patient or the doctor. Some patients, however, may think that the resident is trying to drag out the evaluation to make more money or that the resident is not experienced because the resident is a trainee. These issues and thoughts should be addressed.

As in integrated treatment, the resident should feel in control of the patient's care. Because other clinicians are involved, the resident may sometimes feel like an intruder or a consultant with regard to the case. Although these are honest feelings, one of the key issues in the evaluation is for the resident to feel some ownership over the care of the patient. A tug-of-war over who is in charge, with the patient caught in the middle, is simply unacceptable. The triangulated relationship of therapist, resident, and patient is complicated. Although some might say that the patient is ultimately in charge of care, from a medicolegal standpoint, it is best for the resident to consider himself or herself as being in charge (MacBeth 1999; McNary 2016). In the event of an untoward or untimely death, suicide, or adverse outcome, the physician is usually considered principal care provider (MacBeth 1999; McNary 2016).

Competency

Psychiatry residents must be able to articulate and understand their role in the split/collaborative treatment arrangement: responsibilities, structure, and liabilities.

Split/collaborative treatment can become very complicated for the resident after the initial evaluation is complete. After obtaining information about all aspects of the patient's psychiatric and medical history, the resident must then be able to focus on only a portion of that history (usually medication management) in order to provide the medication component of the split/collaborative treatment. Yet the resident should also always consider the whole patient, especially in relation to the potential for suicide and violence, family issues, and medical problems.

The resident should inform the patient that although certain characteristics will be focused on in treatment, the resident remains interested and concerned about all aspects of the patient's care. The resident should provide the patient with guidelines about when to contact the resident and how to inform him or her of any changes in medical issues or any other adverse events that may or may not be related to medication. In other words, the resident should help the patient understand what issues should be ascribed to the medication and the medical aspects of care and what the patient should do if a situation arises. Many situations related to medication could occur (including side effects and suicidality), so the resident ideally should communicate this information clearly in the initial evaluation.

McNary (2016) suggests that the resident ask the following important questions when providing split/collaborative therapy for a suicidal patient. These are important questions to ask in any split/collaborative therapy arrangement, especially regarding risk management:

1. Who is the patient's therapist, and what are his or her qualifications?
2. How often does the therapist plan on seeing the patient?
3. What gut feelings does the resident have about the therapist (regarding the temperament of the therapist, abilities of the therapist, etc.)?
4. How will the resident and the therapist communicate?
5. Have the resident and the therapist discussed and agreed on their respective roles?
6. Is there a mutual understanding of the patient's current status?
7. How will the resident handle potential conflicts?

Initial Evaluation Outline

The initial psychiatric evaluation should be similar, if not identical, in any treatment arrangement discussed in this book, whether treatment is integrated, split/collaborative *after* referral from a nonmedical therapist or primary care or specialty physician, or split/collaborative *before* referral to a nonmedical therapist or primary care physician. Initial evaluation after a referral from a nonmedical therapist may differ somewhat and may be more difficult.

In this arrangement, the evaluation is colored by information from the referring nonmedical therapist or primary care physician. Ideally, the entire chart is available, and the resident has had time to read the referring note and at least skim through the chart. The evaluation in this situation could be more difficult because of patient transference and resistance to yet another long evaluation. Patients will also unavoidably compare the style and comfort level of the resident with those of the therapist. We emphasize again that it is essential to explain to the patient that the evaluation is going to cover many, if not all, of the issues (and more) that were already discussed in the evaluation with the nonmedical therapist. The reasons for this are that 1) the psychiatrist wants to gain a full understanding of the case and 2) this evaluation is about medication treatment, and some issues might not have been covered in the evaluation by the nonmedical therapist.

In the subsections that follow, we point out the specific issues pertinent to an initial evaluation in split/collaborative treatment after a referral from a nonmedical therapist. Otherwise, the initial evaluation is the same as in integrated treatment.

It is important to note that the order of various components of the initial evaluation may be a matter of personal preference or custom. However, after obtaining basic identifying data, the resident should start with the inquiry about the chief complaint and present illness.

Chief Complaint and Present Illness

In the split/collaborative treatment situation, the outlining of the chief complaint may just repeat the referring clinician's reason for referral (e.g., "The patient was referred for long-standing depression resistant to cognitive-behavioral therapy," or "The patient was referred for a sudden change in behavior and hearing voices during the course of dynamic psychotherapy"). The chief complaint may serve as an introduction to the next part of the evaluation: the present illness.

Questioning about the history of the present illness should start broadly and become more direct and targeted throughout the interview, moving from open-ended questions to targeted questions about symptoms, their onset, possible precipitating factors, impact on functioning, the scope of distress, maladaptive patterns, and other issues. The history of the present illness could also include the psychiatric review of systems (MacKinnon and Yudofsky 1991). Assessment of suicidality and homicidality should be included in this part of the evaluation and should be well documented. Just as in many other areas of questioning, when inquiring about suicidality or homicidally, the resident can mention the referral from the nonmedical therapist. The resident could remark, "Your therapist related to me that you were feeling like harming or killing yourself." Using information obtained from the referring clinician should be done judiciously and carefully, however. The patient may not corroborate this information for various reasons (e.g., no longer feeling suicidal, being afraid of hospitalization, or not trusting the psychiatrist), and pressing the issue could lead to serious transference and resistance. Although the patient may have already been diagnosed by the nonmedical therapist, the resident should not remain focused on only one area of the psychopathology. The resident should establish his or her own possible diagnosis and should always probe other areas of psychopathology (e.g., in depressed patients, ask about anxiety, psychosis).

It is important for the resident to appreciate and manage the emotional content that is offered by the patient at this crucial initial evaluation. Riess (2011) has developed an aid to assist clinicians in becoming more attuned to patients' emotional needs, which may be helpful during training. Evidence shows that during psychotherapeutic encounters, patients and physicians are highly reactive to each other, with physiological correlates of empathy (Del Piccolo and Goss 2012). The resident should try to remain empathetic toward the patient and support the patient's emotional needs.

Psychiatric and Medical Illness History

In this specific situation, the patient's history of psychiatric illness is a very important part of the initial evaluation, because taking a good medical illness history is not always part of the therapist's initial evaluation. This history could have a tremendous impact on treatment planning and selection of treatment modality. A positive response to previous treatment should guide the resident to use the same treatment again, and an unsuccessful treatment trial should guide the resident not to use the same modality again.

The patient should be probed about onset, possible precipitating factors, course, comorbidity, accompanying disability, and treatment. Information about psychiatric hospitalizations should include the patient's age at the time of hospitalization, reason for hospitalization, length of hospitalization, place of hospitalization, what was done during the hospitalization (e.g., medications tried, psychotherapy), the patient's condition at discharge, and the patient's feelings about the hospitalization.

The patient should also be asked about previous treatment. Questions about medications should include the names of the medications, the patient's understanding of the reasons for using a particular medication, the length of treatment with each particular medication, maximum dosages, whether the medication was helpful, what symptoms were relieved the most, and what side effects were present. The patient should also be asked whether he or she is taking any psychotropic medication at the time of the initial evaluation. As Bender and Messner (2003) emphasize, the resident should not assume that the patient is not taking psychotropic medication if he or she is not seeing a psychiatrist. In the split/collaborative treatment arrangement, it is quite important to probe the issue of previous use of medication. It has been our experience that nonmedical therapists frequently do not obtain a good medication history. Similar questions (when, why, what kind, success/failure, patient's feelings about the treatment) should be asked about previous psychotherapy and behavioral therapy. The resident should also ask whether medication was combined with psychotherapy or behavioral therapy in the past.

Previous suicidal thoughts and behavior should be explored and documented, making a distinction between suicidal and self-harming behavior. A thorough exploration of possible substance use history should also occur, with questions specifically asked about alcohol use or misuse and illicit and prescription medication abuse. Patients should be questioned about tobacco and caffeine use as well.

Medical history is another important part of the psychiatric evaluation. The history of serious illnesses and surgeries should be obtained. The resident should consider whether the symptoms with which the patient presents could be a manifestation or reaction to chronic illness. The patient should be asked about medications used to treat any medical conditions, and, preferably, the patient should provide a list of these medications and dosages. Many medications can interfere with the metabolism of psychotropic agents, so this information will be of value to the resident. Female patients should be asked about their menstrual history and should be asked about the possibility of pregnancy before starting medication.

We would like to point out again that a good medical history is usually not obtained by nonmedical therapists. Nonphysicians frequently document medical history by the use of a questionnaire, which may simply list the names of a few diseases without including time frame or treatment documentation. Therefore, the resident needs to conduct a very careful medical history for each patient and not rely on information provided by the referring clinician.

Family History

Information about family history of psychiatric illness and responses to treatment could also have an impact on treatment selection and planning. Family history should include the history of psychiatric and medical illnesses, as well as an exploration of relationships within the family. Information about parents and siblings should be obtained, as well as a history of psychiatric illness and treatment in members of the extended family. The resident should ask specifically about substance abuse and suicide history in family members. The relationships within the family should also be explored, including how the patient gets along with his or her parents and siblings, whether there has been any violence within the family, and whether any emotional neglect or emotional, physical, or sexual abuse has occurred. If asking about physical or sexual abuse, the resident should be sure there is enough time to explore the issue. Waiting until the last few minutes of the evaluation is contraindicated. The resident might handle this by letting the patient know that he or she would like to discuss the issue next time.

Personal and Social History

Personal and social history may help the examining resident with treatment planning in terms of the patient's preferences, family and social support, financial situation, and other factors. The clinician should attempt to elicit a full picture of the patient and his or her life situation starting with the perinatal and developmental history. If time and situation permit, information on developmental milestones, relationships during childhood and adolescence, and emerging personality during childhood and adolescence should be obtained.

Educational history should include information regarding whether the patient graduated from high school (if not, why not and whether a GED [General Educational Development] diploma was obtained), college education, postgraduate education (vs. current employment), and the original educational goals and their fulfillment. The patient should be asked about any history of difficulties at school, either academic or behavioral.

Occupational history should include, if possible, information about all employment, including duration, reason for termination or change, any difficulties at work, and possible exposure to dangerous substances. An important question to consider is whether the patient's employment is commensurate with his or her education level. It is also important to understand if the patient's treatment goals include a change or improvement in occupation or quality of life (Kamenov et al. 2017).

Military history should include the age when the patient was drafted or recruited, reasons for signing up (e.g., idealism, financial reasons, risk and thrill seeking), length of service, deployment, and the nature of and reason for discharge. Military history should also include information about whether the patient experienced combat, sustained any injuries, underwent any disciplinary actions, or was exposed to addictive and/or toxic substances during service. The resident should also ask what it was like returning home, the impact of the patient's service on family, and so forth.

Relational and marital history should include information about any sustained relationships in the patient's life. Inquiry should be made about the age when the patient got married, length of marriage or relationship, past conflicts and disagreements, and present relationship with the partner or spouse. If the patient is divorced, reasons for divorce should be discussed. Information about children—their ages, health, education, and patient's relationship with them—should also be gathered. When the patient presents relational or marital issues as the core of his or her problems, the relational and marital history can be expanded by asking about areas of disagreement, who does what at home, the management of family finances, and relationships with members of the extended family.

Sexual history should include information about psychosexual development, early sexuality, sexual orientation, age at first sexual contact or intercourse, frequency of sexual activity, ability to reach orgasm, any sexual dysfunction (e.g., low libido, erectile dysfunction, lack of lubrication, premature ejaculation, delayed orgasm, anorgasmia, painful orgasm), masturbation, and unusual sexual preferences. We have noted that psychiatric residents frequently omit the sexual history for various reasons, either because they are uncomfortable asking patients about sex or because they are inappropriately worried about offending patients by asking about sexual history. We would like to emphasize that when asked tactfully and in full confidentiality, patients do not usually feel offended by questions about their sexuality and, in fact, appreciate that someone is taking the time to ask about this often-neglected subject.

Some (e.g., MacKinnon and Yudofsky 1991) also suggest asking about *social relationships, friends, religious and cultural background, hobbies, and long-term plans as a part of personal history*. Others (e.g., Bender and Messner 2003, p. 66) recommend obtaining an "adaptive history" by asking questions such as "What stresses have you overcome in the past?"; "How did you do it?"; and "What are your personal strengths?"

Mental Status Examination

The mental status examination is a summary of the physician's observations and the patient's subjective reporting of various areas such as appearance, behavior, feelings, perception, thinking, and cognitive functioning. Most textbooks describe the mental status examination as a long list of categories to be examined at the end of the psychiatric evaluation. An experienced clinician, however, usually begins the mental status examination from the very beginning of the evaluation by observing the patient's appearance and behavior and registering the symptoms that the patient reports. The more formal mental status examination conducted at the end of the psychiatric evaluation should therefore address only areas not previously covered or areas in need of further clarification, such as specific cognitive assessments. The resident should not repeat detailed questioning about symptoms of major depression in a patient who presented with a chief complaint of depressed mood, low energy, poor sleep, and lack of appetite. Instead, the resident might ask about symptoms not mentioned before, such as anhedonia or cognitive impairment.

The mental status examination should include, but not be limited to, the following areas:

- *Attitude and rapport*—Whether the patient comes into the office voluntarily or hesitantly; whether the patient is cooperative, friendly, and appropriate; whether he or she makes eye contact; and the nature of the patient's facial expression.
- *Appearance*—The patient's hygiene, clothing, and special marks (e.g., tattoos).
- *Behavior and psychomotor activity*—The nature of the patient's gait; whether he or she is restless, sits on the edge of the chair, is wringing his or her hands, or has increased motor activity; whether the patient has abnormal movements, tics, dystonias, gesticulations, and so forth. (Some are now including this information in the review of systems in the electronic medical record template.)
- *Speech*—The quantity (e.g., talking all the time or answering only in monosyllabic words) and quality (e.g., errors, tone, rate of production, rhythm) of the patient's speech.
- *Affect*—The expression on the patient's face.
- *Mood and mood congruence/appropriateness and stability (vs. lability)*— "Vegetative" signs, such as sleep (including dreams), appetite, and libido, should be explored. Exploration of this area should also include other symp-

toms of mood disorders, such as possible anhedonia, energy level, and feelings of guilt. The resident should ask about recent suicidal or homicidal ideation and possible plans.

- *Anxiety and related symptoms*—Obsessions, compulsions, panic attacks, worrying, social avoidance, phobias, flashbacks, and startle responses.
- *Perception*—Illusions, hallucinations, and feelings of unreality and depersonalization.
- *Thought process*—Form (e.g., flow of associations, blocking, tangentiality, circumstantiality) and content (e.g., suspiciousness, ideas of reference, thought insertion, delusions—systematized, vague, or isolated—and their content—paranoid or grandiose) of the patient's thought processes; also, in the case of mood disorders, congruency with mood.
- *Alertness and wakefulness.*
- *Orientation*—By time, place, person, and situation.
- *Concentration*—Tested by simple tasks such as serial sevens or spelling certain words forward and backward.
- *Memory*—Recent, intermediate, remote, possible confabulation. Short-term memory and concentration could be tested by asking the patient to remember three things and then asking him or her to recall these things in 5 minutes. (We have observed that many residents do not allow enough time between asking the patient to remember three things and asking for their recollection—asking for recollection almost immediately is meaningless.)
- *Estimate of general information and fund of knowledge*—The patient's ability to provide information about recent events, big cities, famous people, or geography.
- *Estimate of intelligence*—Average, below average, above average; or possible developmental delays.
- *Judgment*—Operational and formal; estimated by asking about reactions to standard situations.
- *Abstraction*—The patient's ability to abstract, which could be tested by asking him or her to interpret proverbs or by discussing similarities and differences.
- *Insight*—The patient's awareness of his or her illness or situation.
- *Impulse control and frustration tolerance.*

Competency

Psychiatry residents should be able to understand and perform a complete psychiatric evaluation of patients who are in split/collaborative treatment arrangements.

Formulation

After finishing the evaluation, the examining resident may briefly formulate the case for himself or herself, considering key issues such as the patient's present illness, past illness, personal history, developmental issues, and ego strengths and defenses. The formulation may be postponed, however, until further information is gathered and any test results have been obtained. In a split/collaborative treatment arrangement, the formulation should primarily rely on the information obtained by the resident but should also take into account information provided by the nonmedical therapist.

Diagnosis

Making the diagnosis (or diagnoses) of the patient by using the multiaxial DSM diagnostic classification (American Psychiatric Association 2000) has been abandoned in the latest edition of DSM (DSM-5; American Psychiatric Association 2013). Many considered the multiaxial diagnosis cumbersome and insufficiently inclusive and considered Axis IV and DSM-IV-TR vague and not very useful. However, we believe that multiaxial diagnosis forces the clinician to consider various areas that may have an impact on treatment planning and treatment outcome, including diagnosis of major mental disorder; possible personality disorder or its traits; intellectual impairment; the presence of physical illness that might be involved in the pathogenesis and that might possibly complicate the treatment planning and outcome; the presence of major stressors; and the level of functioning.

Diagnostic considerations might include decisions about further medical testing, such as a physical examination, laboratory testing (either exploratory, such as thyroid testing for unexplained tiredness and low energy, or as a baseline before starting certain medications, such as liver enzyme testing before beginning certain antipsychotics, or blood urea nitrogen, creatinine, and thyroid tests before starting lithium), measurement of heart rate and blood pressure before starting some medications, possible psychological testing (e.g., memory and other cognitive testing), and neurological examination and other specialized diagnostic testing. The resident might also consider conducting further discussions with the referring nonmedical therapist.

Treatment Planning

In the case of split/collaborative treatment, the initial evaluation is focused on establishing the diagnosis and selecting the most appropriate medication, as well as developing the therapeutic alliance (Del Piccolo and Goss 2012). Both the diagnosis and the treatment selection and plan should be thoroughly discussed with the patient at the end of the initial evaluation (see "Discussion With the Patient/Opening" below). Issues specific to split/collaborative treatment include the patient's relationship with the nonmedical therapist, the nonmedical therapist's attitude toward and relationship with the evaluating psychiatrist, specific insurance regulations (some insurance companies do not allow the patient to be seen by both the psychiatrist and the therapist on the same day), scheduling difficulties for some busy patients (which can result in an additional series of visits), the patient's conscious and unconscious comparison of the psychiatrist and the therapist, and even the gender and ethnicity of both treating parties (e.g., a female patient in treatment for trauma after an assault may see a female nonmedical therapist but may be referred to a male psychiatrist).

To facilitate careful treatment planning, Bender and Messner (2003) suggest organizing psychiatric diagnoses into two categories: 1) disorders with targetable symptoms that meet DSM diagnostic criteria (e.g., mood disorders, anxiety disorders, substance abuse), and 2) conditions more closely linked to ongoing life stressors (e.g., relational problems, occupational problems, adjustment disorders, personality disorders). This distinction may help the resident to make the decision about recommending psychotherapy, medication intervention, or both.

Treatment planning by the resident in a split/collaborative treatment arrangement almost always includes decisions about medication or somatic treatments, such as repetitive transcranial magnetic stimulation or electroconvulsive therapy. In many instances, impairment in daily functioning may be a major decision factor in choosing medication. In the situation in which the patient is referred by a nonmedical therapist for medication treatment, the resident's decision usually includes only medication, unless the evaluating psychiatrist feels that psychotherapy is not indicated or that a different psychotherapy modality should be chosen. Whether or not medication or another somatic treatment is selected, treatment is discussed with the patient (see "Discussion With the Patient/Opening" below), and the patient is referred back to the therapist to continue therapy.

A referral for medication therapy by a nonmedical therapist does not automatically mean that medication is indicated. The nonmedical therapist may be frustrated by a lack of progress in psychotherapy, by unrecognized resistance, or by other issues and may be looking for a path to a more rapid therapeutic response in the form of medication. If the resident feels that medication is not indicated, he or she should explain this to the patient and later discuss this with the referring nonmedical therapist. The reasons for not prescribing medication should be carefully explained and explored during these discussions.

In the situation in which a patient is referred by a nonmedical therapist or is self-referred to the resident and is not in psychotherapy, the resident's decision may include medication, psychotherapy, or both. If the resident believes that medication is not indicated, he or she should decline to prescribe it and explain to the patient the reasoning behind this decision. A conversation with the referring clinician may also be warranted (with the patient's permission). If the resident feels that psychotherapy is indicated in addition to or instead of medication and the resident has no time or is insufficiently qualified to provide the psychotherapy, the resident should refer the patient to a qualified therapist that he or she is familiar with. The decision about selecting the type of psychotherapy could be therapist based (whatever psychotherapy is the therapist's area of expertise), diagnosis based (e.g., cognitive-behavioral therapy for depression or in vivo desensitization for agoraphobia without a history of panic attacks), or outcome based (whatever the goal of therapy is, or whatever could be realistically achieved) (Makover 2016). The resident should contact the therapist to whom he or she is referring the patient, preferably not through an electronic portal.

Discussion With the Patient/Opening

Discussing the diagnosis and the treatment selection and plan with the patient is usually the last step of the initial evaluation (unless the evaluation needs to be extended beyond the first session).

The resident should inform the patient, in simple terms, about the diagnosis and what the diagnosis means in practical terms. The patient should be encouraged to ask questions about the diagnosis and the diagnostic process. The patient should also be informed whether or not the resident agrees with the diagnosis made by the referring nonmedical therapist if applicable. If the resident does not agree with the therapist, he or she should explain why this is.

After discussing the diagnosis, the resident should briefly outline the recommendation for the initial treatment plan. In both kinds of split/collaborative treatment arrangements (a patient referred by a therapist or a new patient), the resident should explain the selection of the medication, what to expect, the time frame (e.g., fairly quick alleviation of anxiety with benzodiazepines vs. 3 weeks waiting for an antidepressant to alleviate depressed mood), and possible side effects and their management. The patient should be also given instructions on how to reach the resident in case there is an emergency or if the patient experiences any bothersome side effects or has any questions. It should be emphasized to the patient that he or she should primarily contact the resident about any issues related to medication or change in clinical status (especially suicidality or homicidality). The availability of the resident often alleviates a lot of the patient's anxiety about starting treatment. It is important to note that some nonmedical therapists cannot be reached in an emergency (i.e., they do not carry a pager and have no answering service) and, as Gitlin and Miklowitz (2016, p. 5) point out, "some routinely tell the patient to page the psychopharmacologist for all urgent situations, even those that are not pharmacologically related."

The patient should also be informed that medication changes could be initiated between appointments over the telephone if necessary (e.g., in case of severely bothersome side effects) but that this is not optimal. As with the diagnosis, patients should be encouraged to ask questions about the treatment. Many patients may have very specific questions based on their Internet searches, direct-to-consumer advertisement, or media reports or sensationalism. Providing medication fact sheets with specific information about side effects can be helpful to some patients; if possible, these should be made available. Some institutions and states require consent forms to be signed by patients or guardians when prescribing psychotropic mediations. Finally, patients should be seen often during the initial phase of treatment with medication, so the patient should be given a follow-up appointment fairly soon. It is simply not acceptable to say, "Here is your prescription; see me in month or two," even if the patient sees his or her therapist somewhat frequently.

If the resident decides that medication is not indicated, this needs to be discussed with the patient. Some patients will be relieved because they are afraid to take medication. Other patients may get angry because they expected a "quick fix," which may not exist. They may feel as if the session with the resident was a waste of time and money. The resident may find that there are other issues (such as substance abuse issues) that should hierarchically be managed first before a psychotropic medication can be prescribed.

In some cases, the patient may be referred for therapy while being started on medication. The resident should explain to the patient why this is the case. Perhaps there is a lack of time in the resident's schedule, an insurance regulation, or perhaps the resident lacks the appropriate expertise.

The initiation of treatment should include summarizing the patient's own perspective of the illness and his or her hopes for treatment. Past experiences with care, including possible negative treatment experiences, are important. There should be discussion of the need for treatment, with inquiry into negative social consequences, and, in the case of pharmacotherapy, comparing mental illness and psychopharmacology to other medical problems and medications, such as diabetes and insulin.

The subsequent sessions during the opening phase of treatment may further deal with issues such as the meaning of medication for the patient; fears related to its value, symptoms, and side effects; the natural tendency to stop treatment when symptoms improve; and benefits and drawbacks of treatment (Beitman et al. 2003).

Pruett and Martin (2003) suggest other issues the resident should be aware of when prescribing medication and combining it with psychotherapy, such as the following:

- The clinician should be constantly aware of the adverse influence of marketing.
- Psychodynamic formulations are essential for evaluating therapeutic alternatives and the effectiveness of combined treatment.
- Residents should actively manage time pressures in meetings with patients, especially in the early appointments.
- The clinician should neither oversell nor undersell any one medication as a part of the treatment regimen but should instead discuss a number of alternatives.

Once the initial evaluation is completed, all information is gathered, and various treatment issues are considered, the resident should discuss the case with the clinical supervisor and the referring therapist or physician.

Discussion With the Referring Therapist or Referring Physician

The final part of the initial evaluation should be to contact the referring nonmedical therapist or primary care physician or the nonmedical therapist to whom the resident is referring the patient. These contacts should be arranged only with the patient's explicit agreement. As noted before, however, HIPAA rules do not apply to communications between treating parties. Some contact with the referral source, at least confirming patient evaluation, should be done. Many institutions require written documentation of the patient's agreement and may have specific forms permitting such contact. The patient not only should be informed that this contact is going to happen but also should have some idea of what will be discussed and whether this will be a one-time contact or (ideally) a long-term arrangement.

The resident may contact the referring therapist or the therapist to whom the patient will be referred in a letter or a written note (sent by regular mail or e-mail); however, personal or telephone contact is preferable. It should be noted in the patient's medical record that this communication occurred and the date and time.

When contacting the therapist who referred the patient, the resident should thank the therapist for the referral and for any information provided. The resident's findings, diagnosis, and treatment decision, as well the treatment plan and further contacts between the resident and the therapist (who, when, in what situation, and why) should be discussed. If medication is not indicated despite the therapist's request, the reasons for not prescribing medication should be carefully and politely discussed. The resident should avoid making premature changes to the treatment based on pressure from the therapist, and, conversely, the resident should avoid criticizing the therapist or making premature suggestions about the therapy.

When contacting the therapist to whom the resident is referring the patient for psychotherapy, the resident should explain the reasons for the referral, plans for medication treatment, further contacts between the resident and patient (who, when, in what situation, and why), and what the resident thinks should be addressed in therapy. This information will help the therapist to understand the case and plan for therapy, regardless of whether the referral is eventually deemed appropriate or not.

References

American Psychiatric Association: Diagnostic and Statistical Manual of Mental Disorders, 4th Edition, Text Revision. Washington, DC, American Psychiatric Association, 2000

American Psychiatric Association: Diagnostic and Statistical Manual of Mental Disorders, 5th Edition. Arlington, VA, American Psychiatric Association, 2013

Beitman BD, Blinder BJ, Thase ME, et al: Integrating Psychotherapy and Pharmacotherapy: Dissolving the Mind-Brain Barrier. New York, WW Norton, 2003

Bender S, Messner E: Becoming a Therapist: What Do I Say, and Why? New York, Guilford, 2003

Del Piccolo L, Goss C: People-centred care: new research needs and methods in doctor-patient communication: challenges in mental health. Epidemiol Psychiatr Sci 21(2):145–149, 2012 22789161

Gitlin MJ, Miklowitz DJ: Split treatment: recommendations for optimal use in the care of psychiatric patients. Ann Clin Psychiatry 28(2):132–137, 2016 27285393

Hansen-Grant S, Riba MB: Contact between psychotherapists and psychiatric residents who provide medication backup. Psychiatr Serv 46(8):774–777, 1995 7583476

Kalman TP, Kalman VN, Granet R: Do psychopharmacologists speak to psychotherapists? A survey of practicing clinicians. Psychodyn Psychiatry 40(2):275–285, 2012 23006119

Kamenov K, Twomey C, Cabello M, et al: The efficacy of psychotherapy, pharmacotherapy and their combination on functioning and quality of life in depression: a meta-analysis. Psychol Med 47(3):414–425, 2017 27780478

MacBeth JE: Divided treatment: legal implications and risks, in Psychopharmacology and Psychotherapy: A Collaborative Approach. Edited by Riba MB, Balon R. Washington, DC, American Psychiatric Press, 1999, pp 111–158

MacKinnon RA, Yudofsky SC: Principles of the Psychiatric Evaluation. Philadelphia, PA, JB Lippincott, 1991

Makover RB: Treatment Planning for Psychotherapists: A Practical Guide to Better Outcomes, 3rd Edition. Washington, DC, American Psychiatric Publishing, 2004

McNary A: Managing the suicidal patient in a split-treatment relationship. Innov Clin Neurosci 13(3–4):42–45, 2016 27354928

Pruett KD, Martin S: Thinking about prescribing: the psychology of psychopharmacology, in Pediatric Psychopharmacology: Principles and Practice. Edited by Martin A, Scahill L, Charney DS, et al. New York, Oxford University Press, 2003, pp 417–425

Riess H: Biomarkers in the psychotherapeutic relationship: the role of physiology, neurobiology, and biological correlates of E.M.P.A.T.H.Y. Harv Rev Psychiatry 19(3):162–174, 2011 21631162

Schen CR, Raymond L, Notman M: Transfer of care of psychotherapy patients: implications for psychiatry training. Psychodyn Psychiatry 41(4):575–595, 2013 24283450

Schofield MJ, Grant J: Developing psychotherapists' competence through clinical supervision: protocol for a qualitative study of supervisory dyads. BMC Psychiatry 13(12), 2013 23298408

Sequencing and Maintenance in Split/Collaborative Treatment

7

Attempting to determine the best way to sequence psychopharmacology and psychotherapy in a split/collaborative treatment arrangement is a real and significant problem (Beitman et al. 2003). Although research has shown that the combination of both types of treatments is effective for patients with many kinds of psychiatric diagnoses (Guidi et al. 2011, 2016) and that the split/collaborative treatment model has become the default paradigm in most clinical organizations (Gitlin and Miklowitz 2016), the research to date has not provided us with a clear guideline for sequencing specific treatments and treatment modalities. Furthermore, the guidelines that do exist based on general considerations of evaluation or treatment of certain types of disorders are focused on integrated treatment, in which a psychiatrist provides both the psychotherapy and medication management (Silverman et al. 2015). Split/collaborative treatment adds other variables that make the logistics and understanding of the sequence more complicated.

Along with the complex nature of sequencing, another complex aspect of treatment is maintenance. Once the patient is stable with medications and some form of psychotherapy, many questions have to be addressed, including how often and for what duration the patient should be seen by each clinician; how often medications should be changed; how often the family should be involved in the sequencing and maintenance phases; when termination should be discussed; and who should be managing the patient's mental health and completing the treatment plans.

It is also important to briefly note the historical backdrop regarding the sequencing of medication and psychotherapy, because it provides a context for the understanding of why this is so difficult. As Roose (2001) explains, in the past there was a hierarchy in the analytic literature of first trying to treat patients with analytic treatment, which would be curative if effective. Medication was used only to relieve symptoms and could be used only if it would not affect the underlying psychic conflicts that were thought to be the origin of the psychological illness. Roose notes that in this context psychotropic medication was equated with inferior medical practice, and it was believed that medication could do significant harm if it masked symptoms enough that the psychiatrist could not determine, and therefore treat, the underlying psychic problems. Medications were to be used by inexperienced therapists and those who were not analytically trained—those who could not engage patients in a long-term dynamic relationship when the real work would be taking place.

The psychodynamic community started to come around to the use of psychotropic medication when research began showing the positive effect of a combination of medication and psychotherapy (Rounsaville et al. 1981; Weissman et al. 1979). By the 1990s, more psychoanalysts were reporting that they were prescribing psychotropic medications for their patients (Donovan and Roose 1995), but by 2000, it seemed that antidepressant medications were possibly still underprescribed by psychodynamic clinicians (Vaughan et al. 2000).

There is probably still a mind–body dualism, in which clinicians ask whether symptoms are biologically driven, whether patients have a "chemical imbalance," whether some symptoms of anxiety and depression would eventually clear without medication, and whether some clinicians medicate too early or too late. These issues are all important, and understanding the history of the field—realizing that some supervisors who are analysts were trained under the mind-body dichotomy—is helpful to the resident and can promote greater understanding. More modern perspectives move beyond the mind–body dualism model, seeing it as reductionistic and insufficiently informed by progress in the clinical neurosciences. Forward-thinking clinical neuroscience embraces psychological processes and underlying biological mechanisms without discarding either "reality." Furthermore, clinical neuroscience holds sacred the traditions of interpersonal healing as well as the highly innovative forms of inquiry that are truly unraveling the mysteries of the brain. Beyond these larger ideological issues, sequencing in split/collaborative care is also more difficult because the resident is not necessarily always involved in the care of the patient from the beginning—that is, from the point when the patient first entered the clinic for the psychiatric evaluation. The patient may have been transferred from one resident to another for psychopharmacology, or the patient may have been referred by a therapist or arrived as a self-referral to see the resident for medication. In either case, the resident will not know what occurred at the beginning of the treatment, what the goals and expectations are for care, or what to do vis-à-vis sequence.

In this chapter, we raise the issues and questions regarding sequencing in split/ collaborative treatment and derive related competencies that could be defined and measured.

What Comes First?

The first task, after performing a good evaluation, is to determine the diagnosis, or at least to have a working multidimensional diagnostic formulation. From the diagnosis, an adequate treatment plan can be developed with consideration of medications or psychotherapy or both.

If the patient is already in psychotherapy with a clinician and is being referred for medication evaluation, then it is up to the resident to determine whether enough information has been obtained to consider providing medication. The most critical questions are the following:

- Does the resident need to obtain more information from the referring therapist or primary care physician?
- Does the resident have information about the patient's past and present medical history and current medications? Has the resident asked the patient about the possibility of pregnancy?
- Has consent for medication been obtained from the patient (if the patient is a minor, from a guardian or parent)?
- Does the patient seem willing to take medication?
- Will the patient be able to have the prescription filled and pay for it and be able to take the medication in a sustained manner?
- Will the patient be able to understand the instructions given regarding the benefits and risks of the medication?
- What are the consequences of not providing medication at this visit?
- When is the next time the patient will be able to return for a follow-up or call to provide feedback?
- Does a supervisor need to hear about the case before the resident prescribes medication? If this is not required, would it be better practice for the resident to obtain supervision?

- Is countertransference on the part of the referring therapist the reason for the referral for a medication evaluation? Is the patient or the therapist feeling frustrated about how the patient's symptoms are being handled in psychotherapy?

Competency

Psychiatry residents should be able to gather enough information to safely prescribe medication in a split/collaborative treatment situation.

If the patient is entering treatment for a psychiatric evaluation and the resident determines that the patient should see another clinician for psychotherapy (i.e., the patient will be in a split/collaborative treatment arrangement), the resident needs to determine whether to prescribe medication at this visit or to wait until the patient has seen the other clinician. Furthermore, the resident needs to work on dynamic and other issues (e.g., transference) and determine whether these issues would affect the type and dosage of medication that would be used. It is also important for the resident to obtain answers to the following questions:

- Does the patient have certain symptoms (e.g., sleep disturbance) that may become worse while waiting for another clinician to see the patient?
- Does the patient have a psychiatric diagnosis (e.g., schizophrenia, major depression) that would make the use of medication at the first visit seem more reasonable than not?
- Does the patient have a personal or family history that suggests medication would be useful?
- Does the patient have a preference or desire for (or, on the contrary, a resistance to) starting medication at the first visit?
- Will it be difficult for the patient to return for a follow-up visit in a short period of time, making it more important to think about medication at the first visit?
- What would be the impact of medication on the patient's performance (at work, etc.), and does the patient possibly need time off from work?
- Does the patient have a suicide/homicide risk, and if so, what is the plan for managing suicidal/homicidal ideation?
- What is the patient's safety network?
- How much medication should be safely provided?

Competency

Psychiatry residents should be able to determine the factors that might make it judicious to provide medication at the first visit.

Although "split" may be a more apt description of the split/collaborative treatment arrangement from the resident's perspective, the patient should feel that the treatment is collaborative and that the care is integrated and unified. It is therefore important for the resident to understand that although there are at least two clinicians providing the psychiatric care, the patient should perceive the care as being seamless.

What Comes Next?

Assuming that the resident decides to provide medication to the patient at the first visit, what should follow is outlined below:

- The resident needs to determine what the major side effects of providing medication could be, what information regarding side effects should be given to the patient, and what the provision for management should be if side effects occur (e.g., should the patient call the resident or discontinue medication). We recommend that the resident consider asking the patient to call the resident between the first and second appointments to relay how he or she is doing with the medication.
- The patient should be instructed to call the resident between psychiatric appointments if any changes occur regarding other medications or physical conditions (e.g., being prescribed a new antihypertensive medication).
- The resident should make sure that consent is obtained from the patient to send copies of the evaluation, including medication information, to the referring clinician and to other medical clinicians involved in the patient's care (e.g., cardiologist).
- Although all follow-up psychiatric notes do not necessarily have to go to the outside clinicians (e.g., cardiologist) and to the therapist, the resident needs to have some regular communication with these clinicians regarding medical issues (such as medication and safety).
- If medication is prescribed, we recommend that the resident have the patient bring a close significant other to a future meeting in order to discuss any issues the family member might have, especially regarding medication.
- Thorough medical records should be kept and should include what the resident has told the patient regarding side effects, time course of medication, and so forth.
- If there is such a requirement by the local or state authorities, the consent to take psychotropic medication should be completed by the patient and placed in the patient's chart.
- The resident should ask the patient how best to prescribe the medication: for example, some patients send away for larger supplies of medication (e.g., 90 days) to cut down on their copayment; some managed care companies

require certain types and dosages of medication to be prescribed; and some managed care companies require preauthorization of medications, particularly those that are not on their formulary.

- The resident should discuss whether any small children live in the home and how to keep the medication safely out of their reach.

Competency

Psychiatry residents should be able to demonstrate that appropriate members of the patient's clinical team will know what medical care and medications are being recommended or provided by the resident.

What If Medication Is Not Prescribed?

If a therapist or other clinician refers the patient to the resident and the resident decides *not* to provide medication, what does this mean to the patient and the referring clinician?

There could be an expectation on the part of the patient that medication is the answer to the patient's problems and symptoms. The patient could be quite disappointed, therefore, if the resident does not see the need to medicate. The patient might be disappointed that he or she had to pay for an evaluation that resulted in "no treatment," because the patient might only value this type of evaluation when it results in a prescription. If there is no basis for a biological etiology for the patient's symptoms, the patient may have to be given a different degree of responsibility in treatment (Gitlin and Miklowitz 2016).

On the basis of what the resident observes in the initial appointment, the resident might disagree with the referring clinician's diagnosis but remain unsure about the need for medication. The resident might tell the patient that although there does not seem to be a need for medication now, but judgment will be reserved until future sessions.

The patient might be pleased that medication is not being provided. The patient might not have wanted to take medication anyway (perhaps because he or she is frightened of taking medication) and may be relieved that it is not going to be prescribed. Furthermore, not having to take medication also means that the cost of treatment will potentially be lower.

Family members or significant others might also have expectations about medication and what it means if the resident does not prescribe. They might have had strong hopes that medication would quickly solve the patient's problems, and these hopes might be dashed when the resident does not prescribe. On the other hand, family members may also have negative feelings about medication, which they may have conveyed to the patient openly or secretly.

Countertransference issues are often involved when a therapist recommends that a patient be seen for medication evaluation. The patient may have many questions about the situation: Why is the evaluation being ordered at this time? What kinds of symptoms are frustrating the therapist? Why can't the therapist fix the problems with psychotherapy alone? What does this mean with regard to the diagnosis? Was the therapist not doing a good enough job? Did the therapist miss something in the ongoing psychiatric care that led to the medication evaluation? What does it mean to get another clinician (the psychiatry resident) involved in the care?

The resident should make sure that he or she is getting the supervision needed to best understand the dynamics of this complex situation. Often, these types of split/collaborative treatment cases are not supervised by the long-term supervisor (who tends to supervise only one or two cases); the general outpatient supervisor tends to just go over the problem cases or the cases that the resident brings to his or her attention. Split/collaborative cases are often overlooked in the supervisory process because on the surface—particularly if there is no medication involved—they seem to pose no problem. These types of cases are truly the most worrisome, however, because of issues and questions that might have been overlooked in the interview, problems that the patient might have been masking, or the inexperience of the resident. Thus, we recommend that training programs assign supervisors expressly to help residents deal with the issues specific to integrated and split/collaborative treatment arrangements. More research needs to be done in this area of clinical supervision (Schofield and Grant 2013).

If medication is not prescribed at the first session, the resident might ask the patient to come back in a few weeks for a reassessment. Often patients, like anyone else, present differently at different times. The resident could view this kind of arrangement as an extended evaluation or an evaluation with a follow-up. This gives the resident another chance to review the symptoms, to think about the patient in the interim, and to determine whether the original diagnosis and treatment plan should stand. This also gives the patient the opportunity to think about whether they want to return to see the resident, to think about what it means to receive medication, and to talk with their therapist about this issue.

There is a great deal of pressure on the resident to get out the prescription pad or computer (for electronic prescribing) and write a prescription for the patient at the initial visit. Under these circumstances, it is probably easier to write a prescription than not to write one. The resident should not feel pressured by the expectations of the patient, the family member, or the referring therapist if the resident does not feel that medication is indicated. Factors more important than other's preferences need to be taken into account, including the patient's symptoms and past psychiatric history, such as suicidal history (or self-harm) and current suicidal symptoms, and personality structure, such as borderline personality disorder. Indeed, there are increased risk management concerns in managing the suicidal patient in split/collaborative treatment relationship (McNary 2016).

Competency

Psychiatry residents must be able to determine when not to prescribe medication in a split/collaborative treatment arrangement.

If Medication Is Prescribed, How Often and What Kind of Collaborative Process Should Be Arranged for the Patient?

With any patient, once medication has been started, it is usually a good idea to see the patient more often than usual until the psychiatric symptoms have stabilized and any untoward side effects can be minimized. This process might require that the patient be seen every 2–3 weeks or even more frequently at the beginning of pharmacotherapy. Telephone calls or e-mails between sessions could also be used. We recommend that the first follow-up visit take place within 1 week if possible. Having frequent visits during the initial phase of treatment not only can be useful in the management of side effects but also can help in building the doctor–patient relationship and in overcoming the patient's disappointment with the delayed onset of action of some medications.

Because it is difficult for the patient to remember exactly what was said during the visit, the psychiatry resident should write down instructions for taking medications. Most emergency rooms and inpatient units provide written instructions for patients, as do many general medical and surgical clinics. It is a good idea for the resident either to type the instructions for dosing, side effects, and so on for each patient or to have preprinted forms on which the pertinent instructions can be checked off. Some clinics or electronic medical record smart sets have such forms available for use. This type of instruction should be made a routine part of each visit.

It should be made clear to patients whom they should call when new symptoms develop. For example, if a patient starts to have suicidal feelings after beginning to take an antidepressant, should he or she call the therapist or the resident? We urge psychiatry residents to ask their patients to let them know when such feelings arise. The resident should also ask the patient to convey to his or her therapist that the resident wants to be told about any suicidal, homicidal, or violent feelings that the patient develops. When such symptoms develop, the patient should of course be seen promptly by a medical professional, which might include asking the patient to go to an emergency room.

It is important to talk with patients about when certain symptoms might be alleviated (weeks vs. days) and what to expect if the symptoms are not relieved (perhaps an increase in dosage, a change in the time of dosing, the addition of an adjunctive medication, or a change in medications).

It is a standard tenet in medicine to do one thing at a time so that the effect of the change on the condition can be observed. If the patient is already in psychotherapy or begins receiving psychotherapy at some point during the time medication is prescribed, then it is very hard to control for the effects of the medication versus the effect of the combined medication and psychotherapy. As Roose (2001) notes, "[T]here has been to date no systematic study of combining medication with psychodynamic psychotherapies" (p. 45). It is therefore almost impossible for the clinicians and the patient to determine the cause and effect of any changes or the full impact of either psychotherapy or medication when they are combined. Therefore, the clinicians have to work very hard with each other and with the patient to determine if the combination is having an impact on the patient and whether that impact is positive or negative.

Although we have avoided referring to specific diagnoses, we would like to point out that a split/collaborative treatment situation could be especially difficult for patients with borderline personality disorder or other Cluster B personality disorders. As Gabbard (2001) points out, many patients with personality disorders are currently treated with a combination of medication and psychotherapy, although the scientific evidence for this approach is limited and most of this treatment is based on clinical impressions that patients with personality disorders have better outcomes with this combination than with either treatment modality alone. Various medications and therapies have been used and combined for patients with personality disorders, with the choices of medication frequently depending on the target symptoms (e.g., neuroleptics for cognitive-perceptual symptoms; antidepressants for affective and mood symptoms; and selective serotonin reuptake inhibitors, mood stabilizers, and other medications for impulsive-behavioral symptoms). There is some evidence that combined treatment of psychotherapy and pharmacotherapy may be beneficial in the treatment of borderline personality disorder (Bozzatello and Bellino 2016).

Combining treatment modalities is almost a rule for Cluster B personality disorders. These patients frequently end up in resident-staffed clinics and in split/collaborative treatment. In the split/collaborative treatment setting, many of these patients tend to play care providers against each other by disparaging one care provider to the other. Patients may idealize the prescribing physician and devalue the therapist or vice versa (Gabbard 2001). In resident-staffed clinics, these patients may also idealize the *previous* prescribing resident (alone or together with the therapist) and demonize the resident who has just assumed their care. Such patients, for example, may demand more time for pharmacotherapy appointments, arguing that the therapist spends more time with them (or the previous resident spent more time with them) and cares more about them. As Gabbard illustrates, these patients might also demand that the omnipotent resident rescue them from the neglectful treatment provided by the nonprescribing therapist. This pattern of behavior is called *splitting,* which may add to the confusion of terminology. In discussing risk management and treatment of the suicidal patient in a split/collaborative treatment relationship, McNary (2016) calls this a "split in split treatment."

As Gabbard (2001) pointed out long ago, this type of splitting is inherent to borderline personality disorder and cannot be entirely prevented or avoided. There are, however, several measures that could be taken to minimize the destructive impact of splitting on the treatment process. These measures should be made very clear to the patient at the beginning of both treatment modalities (pharmacotherapy and psychotherapy) and also whenever a new resident takes over the case.

The first measure is frequent communication and consultation between the care providers. The second measure is ensuring that certain limits specific to the case are established and discussed with both the patient and the care providers at the onset of treatment (either—preferably—with all parties together or with each separately). Examples include limiting the discussion of medication and side effects only to the medication reviews with the psychiatrist and limiting the use of telephone calls and e-mails to each care provider. Finally, as Gabbard (2001, p. 89) suggests, both care providers should agree that "when the patient begins to disparage one of the treaters, the clinician who receives the information should contact the other treater to discuss what is going on rather than acting on the information given by the patient." If the patient does not agree with these rules up front, the resident should probably not agree to treat the patient (Gabbard 2001).

Although the split/collaborative treatment arrangement seems to provide a basis for splitting in patients with borderline personality disorder, this treatment arrangement may also provide some advantages. As Gabbard (2001) notes, the intensity of transference may be diluted by having two care providers in split/collaborative treatment; the patient cannot avoid psychotherapeutic issues by focusing on medication (as could happen in integrated treatment), and care providers may gain insight from one another because they have different perspectives.

How Should Medication Changes Be Addressed?

The psychiatry resident sees the patient at least every 2–3 weeks for medication adjustments, while at the same time the patient is seeing another therapist for psychotherapy. It is very important that the resident and the clinician talk to each other to determine the impact of the medication on the psychotherapy. Is the patient staying engaged in the psychotherapy? Is the patient upset over being sent to the psychiatry resident for medication? Does the patient feel annoyed about having to see two clinicians, paying for two clinicians' time, and worrying about whether there is communication between them? It is important that the patient does not become a "monkey in the middle," that is, the communicator between the resident and the therapist. Communication between the resident and the therapist needs to be worked out at the beginning of care. The patient should be apprised of this communication and the method of communication.

In this kind of split/collaborative arrangement, residents often feel pressured to make medication changes. If the patient is not being seen very often, the resident might be inclined to make changes (e.g., increase dosages, switch too quickly to another type of medication, or add a new medication to the regimen) whenever he or she next sees the patient. If the resident starts feeling pressured to do this, he or she should consider seeing the patient more often or asking the patient to call between visits to talk about medication issues.

What Constitutes Maintenance in Split/Collaborative Treatment?

What constitutes maintenance in a split/collaborative treatment arrangement, especially when some of the symptoms are related to psychic conflicts? Is the alleviation of all symptoms the goal of medication?

At the beginning of treatment, it is important for the resident, the therapist, and the patient to determine the goal of medication in order to avoid undermedicating or overmedicating. If sleep is the target symptom, the goal of the medication might be to ensure that the patient is able to fall asleep in a reasonable time and stay asleep in order not to feel somnolent during the day, to be able to work, and so forth. Similarly, if the goal is for the patient to have no depressive symptoms, then other aspects of the patient's life—such as employment or marital difficulties, or substance use issues—might need to be modified before medications are changed.

Self-report measures, such as the Beck Depression Inventory, are sometimes useful to permit patients to monitor themselves regularly and determine where they are on a symptom checklist. This helps give the patient and the clinician a reference point and allows them to talk about the specific issues that might be getting in the way of the full resolution of the patient's psychiatric problems.

During the maintenance phase, it is a good idea to talk about termination. What is the end point of the split/collaborative treatment? The termination should be sequenced, with the medication and the psychotherapy being completed at separate times. The decision regarding termination should be a mutual agreement between the patient, the therapist, and the psychiatry resident.

If the resident is going to be rotating off the service or graduating, this is also considered a termination with the resident, although it is not necessarily a termination of treatment. Many junior residents do not appreciate the importance of their work with patients and therefore try to minimize the significance of the termination that comes with graduation. They may broach the issue just when they are about to leave without giving the patients enough warning or enough time to process the loss (Schen et al. 2013). Residents might feel bad about leaving, as if they were abandoning their patients.

It is important to try to match patients up with each resident instead of handing the next resident an entire list of patients. Patients want to know who they will be seeing and why they are being assigned to that particular resident. They want to know if there will be a proper sign-off (sometimes called "warm handoff"), if they will need to tell their entire story again to the next resident, etc. These terminations ideally should be discussed during the maintenance phase, and proper time and attention should be paid to this important issue, especially regarding appropriate education, training, and supervision.

Competency

Psychiatry residents should be able to demonstrate knowledge that the issues of maintenance in split/collaborative treatment include termination issues.

The issues of termination are discussed in detail in Chapter 9 "Termination in Integrated and Split/Collaborative Treatment."

Conclusion

Sequencing of pharmacotherapy and psychotherapy in split/collaborative treatment is very difficult. Many patient variables, diagnostic issues, and communication patterns between the referring clinician and the therapist need to be worked out, and there are as yet no clear guidelines based on evidence-based research.

Furthermore, if multiple patients are being cared for in this kind of arrangement, there are often several therapists for the psychiatry resident to communicate with, resulting in increased time and workload. Furthermore, there may be increased risks associated with caring for suicidal patients and those with borderline personality disorder in a split/collaborative treatment arrangement. The task of working with so many clinicians and patients with variable and complex psychiatric conditions is quite difficult and taxing.

We recommend that supervisors and training directors take particular heed of this last point. To the extent possible, we recommend that training programs not ask residents to have so many patients in split/collaborative treatment with so many different therapists that the resident cannot develop a good working relationship with each therapist of every patient they see. Although we understand that this situation often occurs in private practice, it is neither optimal nor acceptable to place residents in such a difficult situation during training. Furthermore, the case mix and the risk management aspects of the case mix should be reviewed by supervisors and training directors and with the residents.

We also recommend that residents be provided good supervision on their split/collaborative treatment cases, especially during the beginning of each case, during maintenance, and when termination is discussed. It is hard for patients to terminate treatment with their doctors, and inexperienced residents often do not appreciate, or do not want to appreciate, the strong transference feelings that patients develop, even in a short time, with residents nor the countertransference feelings that the residents have engendered.

It is also sometimes very useful to have ongoing group supervision of residents, using seminars structured around case conferences and clinical material to help incorporate the principles of both psychotherapy and pharmacotherapy. Novel workshops such as the Psychopharmacology Prescribing Workshops developed by Columbia University, Yale University, and New York University departments of psychiatry are very interesting and could be used as models (Kavanagh et al. 2017).

References

Beitman BD, Blinder BJ, Thase ME, et al: The sequencing problem (using panic disorder as an example), in Integrating Psychotherapy and Pharmacotherapy: Dissolving the Mind-Brain Barrier. New York, WW Norton, 2003, pp 85–103

Bozzatello P, Bellino S: Combined therapy with interpersonal psychotherapy adapted for borderline personality disorder: a two-years follow-up. Psychiatry Res 240:151–156, 2016 27107668

Donovan SJ, Roose SP: Medication use during psychoanalysis: a survey. J Clin Psychiatry 56(5):177–178, discussion 179, 1995 7737955

Gabbard GO: Combining medication with psychotherapy in the treatment of personality disorders, in Psychotherapy for Personality Disorders. Edited by Gunderson JG, Gabbard GO (Review of Psychiatry Series; Oldham JM and Riba MB, series eds). Washington, DC, American Psychiatric Publishing, 2001, pp 65–94

Gitlin MJ, Miklowitz DJ: Split treatment: recommendations for optimal use in the care of psychiatric patients. Ann Clin Psychiatry 28(2):132–137, 2016 27285393

Guidi J, Fava GA, Fava M, et al: Efficacy of the sequential integration of psychotherapy and pharmacotherapy in major depressive disorder: a preliminary meta-analysis. Psychol Med 41(2):321–331, 2011 20444307

Guidi J, Tomba E, Fava GA: The sequential integration of pharmacotherapy and psychotherapy in the treatment of major depressive disorder: a meta-analysis of the sequential model and a critical review of the literature. Am J Psychiatry 173(2):128–137,
2016 26481173

Kavanagh EP, Cahill J, Arbuckle MR, et al: Psychopharmacology prescribing workshops:
a novel method for teaching psychiatry residents how to talk with patients abut medications. Acad Psychiatry, February 13, 2017 [Epub ahead of print] 28194682

McNary A: Managing the suicidal patient in a split-treatment relationship. Innov Clin
Neurosci 13(3–4):42–45, 2016 27354928

Roose SP: Psychodynamic therapy and medication: can treatments in conflict be integrated?
in Integrated Treatment of Psychiatric Disorders. Edited by Kay J (Review of Psychiatry Series; Oldham JM and Riba MB, series eds). Washington, DC, American
Psychiatric Publishing, 2001, pp 31–50

Rounsaville BJ, Klerman GL, Weissman MM: Do psychotherapy and pharmacotherapy
for depression conflict? Empirical evidence from a clinical trial. Arch Gen Psychiatry
38(1):24–29, 1981 7006556

Schen CR, Raymond L, Notman M: Transfer of care of psychotherapy patients: implications for psychiatry training. Psychodyn Psychiatry 41(4):575–595, 2013 24283450

Schofield MJ, Grant J: Developing psychotherapists' competence through clinical supervision: protocol for a qualitative study of supervisory dyads. BMC Psychiatry
13:12, 2013 23298408

Silverman JJ, Galanter M, Jackson-Triche M, et al; American Psychiatric Association:
The American Psychiatric Association Practice Guidelines for the Psychiatric
Evaluation of Adults. Am J Psychiatry 172(8):798–802, 2015 26234607

Vaughan SC, Marshall RD, Mackinnon RA, et al: Can we do psychoanalytic outcome research? A feasibility study. Int J Psychoanal 81 (Pt 3):513–527, 2000 10967773

Weissman MM, Prusoff BA, Dimascio A, et al: The efficacy of drugs and psychotherapy
in the treatment of acute depressive episodes. Am J Psychiatry 136(4B):555–558,
1979 371421

Evaluation, Monitoring, and Supervision of Integrated and Split/Collaborative Treatment

8

The aim of graduate medical education is to form physicians who can provide care expertly and compassionately—in short, to produce competent physicians. In the preceding chapters, we discussed how to acquire the necessary skills to become competent in planning and delivering integrated and split/collaborative treatment. But how does one ensure that the educational process is heading in the right direction and that psychiatry residents will accrue and ultimately possess the required skills and knowledge to competently practice integrated and split/collaborative treatment? Residents' progress in acquiring these skills and knowledge sets has to be adequately and appropriately supervised, monitored, assessed, and evaluated. Competency has to be properly documented, not only because the Review Committee and the program reviewers will be looking for the ways competency is documented in each area but also because properly constructed documentation of the process will allow training programs to appropriately structure the educational process and address deficiencies and other issues requiring improvement or correction.

As Scheiber and Kramer (2003, p. 4) note:

> Competence is not an all-or-nothing proposition. Competence is measured along a sliding scale through demonstrated knowledge and performed tasks. Competence is assessed by degrees. The measuring of medical competence has been a difficult activity. Just how much and exactly what must a physician know and be able to do to be judged "competent"?

What It Means to Be Competent

The first important question is, What does it means to be competent? In general, being *competent* means being well qualified, capable, and "having requisite or adequate abilities or qualities" (Merriam-Webster and 2003, p. 253). It also means being qualified or fit to perform a certain activity. Although being competent requires a certain level of expertise, it is not the same as being an expert. Most educators emphasize that being competent means achieving a skill level approximately midway between that of a novice or dilettante and that of an expert. The concept of defining, teaching, and evaluating or measuring competence (or competencies) is relatively new to medicine in general and to psychiatry in particular. Valid and reliable assessments are elusive, because there is little consensus in the field on exactly what it means to be competent in certain areas and the operational definitions of what it means to be competent are slowly evolving (Guerrero et al. 2017). We suggest that being competent in integrated or split/collaborative treatment means being qualified, knowledgeable, and skillful in integrating and combining two important treatment approaches (pharmacotherapy and various psychotherapies). It also means being knowledgeable about and skillful in providing these two treatments separately and in the context of other forms of medical care, including subspecialized psychiatric care. In addition, being competent in split/collaborative treatment means being skillful and capable in collaborating with other professionals in team-based clinical care settings.

Combined Pharmacotherapy and Psychotherapy Competency Standards and Domains

Most of the authors and working groups that address the evaluation of competencies, including the Royal College of Psychiatrists, suggest focusing on three domains of competency in various psychotherapies: knowledge, skills, and attitudes.

We chose to present the reader with two ways of summarizing the issues of competency in combined pharmacotherapy and psychotherapy. First, we provide the list of proposed competency standards related to integrated and split/collaborative treatment as they appear in this book. Second, we summarize the competency issues according to the three domains: knowledge, skills, and attitudes. This brief summary could be used to create an assessment and evaluation form.

Proposed Competency Standards Related to the Discussion in This Book

Competencies Related to Integrated Treatment

1. Psychiatry residents should demonstrate an appreciation for the triage system that is in place at their institution for both inpatient and outpatient psychotherapy and psychopharmacological treatments (Chapter 1, "Introduction to Integrated and Split/Collaborative Treatment").
2. Psychiatry residents should be able to demonstrate the ability to take a history regarding factors that would influence the decision to provide the patient with split/collaborative versus integrated treatment (Chapter 1, "Introduction to Integrated and Split/Collaborative Treatment").
3. Psychiatry residents should be able to demonstrate the ability to ask questions regarding why the patient is being seen for a psychiatric evaluation (potentially for medication and psychotherapy) (Chapter 2, "Selection of Medication and Psychotherapy in Integrated Treatment").
4. At the initial outpatient session, psychiatry residents must demonstrate the ability to establish a doctor–patient relationship and to provide a trusting, warm environment to explore the patient's needs and problems. Psychiatry residents must be able to discuss medication properly and explain possible side effects and complications (Chapter 2, "Selection of Medication and Psychotherapy in Integrated Treatment").
5. During the evaluation phase, psychiatry residents must be able to demonstrate the ability to develop a biopsychosocial formulation of the patient's problems, develop a problem list, and, together with the patient, develop treatment aims and prioritize problems. Residents must be able to explain to the patient what treatment is being used and why the treatment is appropriate (Chapter 2, "Selection of Medication and Psychotherapy in Integrated Treatment").
6. Psychiatry residents should, based on their evaluation of the patient and their preliminary diagnosis, be able to select the appropriate pharmacotherapy or psychotherapy, or combination (Chapter 3, "Evaluation and Opening in Integrated Treatment").

7. Psychiatry residents should be able to discuss with and explain to the patient the selection of treatment modalities and their rationale (Chapter 3, "Evaluation and Opening in Integrated Treatment").

8. Psychiatry residents must be able to demonstrate the ability to form a working therapeutic alliance at the beginning of treatment (Chapter 4, "Sequencing in Integrated Treatment").

9. Psychiatry residents must be able to demonstrate the ability to appreciate the issues that involve sequencing of medication (and/or other medical treatments) and psychotherapy (Chapter 4, "Sequencing in Integrated Treatment").

10. Psychiatry residents must be able to demonstrate knowledge of the factors that are important for the individual patient to maintain and adhere to a treatment regimen (Chapter 4, "Sequencing in Integrated Treatment").

Competencies Related to Split/Collaborative Treatment

1. Psychiatry residents must be able to determine under what conditions split/collaborative treatment would be most appropriate for a patient and must be able to convey these issues to the patient (Chapter 5, "Selection of Medication, Psychotherapy, and Clinicians in Split/Collaborative Treatment").

2. Psychiatry residents should be able to demonstrate the ability to determine their role in a split/collaborative treatment arrangement and to obtain the appropriate information from the patient, medical records, the referring therapist, other medical clinicians, family members, and other sources (Chapter 5, "Selection of Medication, Psychotherapy, and Clinicians in Split/Collaborative Treatment").

3. Psychiatry residents should develop the ability to potentially reformulate a case (Chapter 5, "Selection of Medication, Psychotherapy, and Clinicians in Split/Collaborative Treatment").

4. Psychiatry residents need to demonstrate how best to terminate psychotherapy when both psychotherapy and pharmacotherapy are provided (Chapter 5, "Selection of Medication, Psychotherapy, and Clinicians in Split/Collaborative Treatment").

5. Psychiatry residents must be able to understand the various dynamic and biological reasons for the request for a psychopharmacological consultation and must be able to obtain the appropriate information to make an informed decision about the diagnosis and treatment plan (Chapter 6, "Evaluation and Opening in Split/Collaborative Treatment").

6. Psychiatry residents should be able to determine the multiple issues that need to be addressed in the initial evaluation of a patient being referred by an outside therapist or physician or as a self-referral (Chapter 6, "Evaluation and Opening in Split/Collaborative Treatment").

7. Psychiatry residents must be able to balance the number of patients in split/collaborative treatment with the complex and time-consuming nature of evaluating and treating such patients (Chapter 6, "Evaluation and Opening in Split/Collaborative Treatment").

8. Psychiatry residents must be able to articulate and understand their role in the split/collaborative treatment arrangement: responsibilities, structure, and liabilities (Chapter 6, "Evaluation and Opening in Split/Collaborative Treatment").

9. Psychiatry residents should be able to understand and perform a complete psychiatric evaluation of patients who are in split/collaborative treatment arrangements (Chapter 6, "Evaluation and Opening in Split/Collaborative Treatment").

10. Psychiatry residents should be able to gather enough information to safely prescribe medication in a split/collaborative treatment situation (Chapter 7, "Sequencing and Maintenance in Split/Collaborative Treatment").

11. Psychiatry residents should be able to determine the factors that might make it judicious to provide medication at the first visit (Chapter 7, "Sequencing and Maintenance in Split/Collaborative Treatment").

12. Psychiatry residents should be able to demonstrate that appropriate members of the patient's clinical team will know what medical care and medications are being recommended or provided by the resident (Chapter 7, "Sequencing and Maintenance in Split/Collaborative Treatment").

13. Psychiatry residents must be able to determine when not to prescribe medication in a split/collaborative treatment arrangement (Chapter 7, "Sequencing and Maintenance in Split Treatment").

14. Psychiatry residents should be able to demonstrate knowledge that the issues of maintenance of split/collaborative treatment include termination issues (Chapter 7, "Sequencing and Maintenance in Split/Collaborative Treatment").

15. Psychiatry residents should be able to demonstrate the factors that are helpful in terminating care with patients (Chapter 9, "Termination in Integrated and Split/Collaborative Treatment").

16. Psychiatry residents should be able to demonstrate the skills and knowledge to terminate pharmacotherapy with a patient when both pharmacotherapy and psychotherapy were provided by the resident (Chapter 9, "Termination in Integrated and Split/Collaborative Treatment").

17. Psychiatry residents should be able to demonstrate the skills and knowledge to terminate psychotherapy with a patient when both pharmacotherapy and psychotherapy were provided by the resident (Chapter 9, "Termination in Integrated and Split/Collaborative Treatment").

18. Psychiatry residents should be able to demonstrate the skills and knowledge to terminate both pharmacotherapy and psychotherapy with a patient when

both pharmacotherapy and psychotherapy were provided by the resident (Chapter 9, "Termination in Integrated and Split/Collaborative Treatment").

19. Psychiatry residents should become familiar with various technologies (e.g., telepsychiatry) through which they can consult with the primary care team (Chapter 10, "Primary Care and Split/Collaborative Care: Improving Access, Decreasing Costs, Improving Outcomes").

20. Psychiatry residents should be able to provide consultation regarding patients with a comorbid severe mental disorder and physical illness, such as diabetes mellitus or hypertension (Chapter 10, "Primary Care and Split/Collaborative Care: Improving Access, Decreasing Costs, Improving Outcomes").

21. Psychiatry residents should be able to discuss with the primary care physician issues such as the goals and expected outcome of psychiatric consultation/treatment, difficulties in communication, the management of side effects, the fostering of adherence, the roll of psychotherapy, and the joint effort to promote a healthy lifestyle for the patient (Chapter 10, "Primary Care and Split/Collaborative Care: Improving Access, Decreasing Costs, Improving Outcomes").

These standards should provide residents, supervisors, and training directors with guidelines for thinking about, learning, teaching, and supervising competency in combined pharmacotherapy and psychotherapy treatment. The reader can quickly refer to the text to which each standard relates.

Competency Domains for Combined Pharmacotherapy and Psychotherapy

To be most helpful to residents and psychiatric educators, we have organized this section based on the template of the competency domains—knowledge, skills, and attitudes—for psychotherapy and psychopharmacology developed by the American Association of Directors of Psychiatry Residency Training (Sargent et al. 2001).

Knowledge

At the end of training, the psychiatry resident should demonstrate understanding and knowledge of the following:

1. Diagnoses and clinical conditions that warrant consideration of psychopharmacological treatment in addition to psychotherapy, or psychotherapy in addition to psychopharmacology.

2. Different methods of combining psychotherapy and psychopharmacology (i.e., integrated and split/collaborative treatment).

3. Specific indications for a recommendation of psychotherapy and psychopharmacology and the ability to determine which type of psychotherapy and medication is warranted.
4. Potential synergies and antagonisms in combining pharmacotherapy and psychotherapy.
5. The multiple psychological and sociocultural meanings that taking medication may have to a patient.
6. The background, education, and training of other mental health professionals who may provide psychotherapy in a combined treatment regimen.
7. Medicolegal and psychotherapeutic issues in the context of one clinician prescribing medication and another providing psychotherapy, including confidentiality, informed consent, and collaboration.
8. The necessity of continuing education in combined pharmacotherapy and psychotherapy for further skill development.
9. The comorbidity of mental illness and substance abuse with serious physical illness and the possible complications when treating these comorbidities and combining various psychotropic and nonpsychotropic medications.

Skills

At the end of training, the psychiatry resident should demonstrate understanding and knowledge of how to carry out the following:

1. Integrate biological and psychological aspects of a patient's history with other clinically relevant information to assess the need for, recommend, and implement pharmacotherapy or psychotherapy in integrated or split/collaborative treatment, either sequentially or simultaneously, in a mutually beneficial manner.
2. Complete the assessment for medication within the context of a psychotherapeutic framework while making interpretations and empathic comments.
3. Form an active alliance with the patient that facilitates adherence with both pharmacotherapy and psychotherapy.
4. Understand how the meaning of a medication to a patient can significantly affect its efficacy and learn how to explore the psychological and sociocultural meanings of medication to a patient.
5. Appreciate the potential psychodynamic issues of prescribing medication (resistance, compliance, and transitional object).
6. Use the placebo effect to prescribe medication more successfully.
7. Provide psychoeducation about medication in a manner that complements the chosen psychotherapy, appreciating the limitations of each treatment modality.

8. Identify and address the psychological aspects of nonadherence with medication regimens.
9. Use transference and countertransference and other psychotherapy techniques while prescribing medication to diminish resistance to medication and facilitate its use when appropriate.
10. Monitor the patient's condition and modify the pharmacotherapy or psychotherapy approach when necessary.
11. Appreciate and assess the importance of timing in pharmacotherapy and psychotherapy interventions.
12. Recognize the ways that prescribing medication can enhance or hinder psychotherapy and the ways that psychotherapy can enhance or hinder pharmacotherapy.
13. Recognize and identify affects in the patient and in himself or herself.
14. Assess suicidality/homicidality on an ongoing basis as it relates to the prescribed medication (or medications).
15. Manage the termination process in both integrated and split/collaborative treatment.
16. Recognize the patient's splitting between the resident and psychotherapist and address it in an appropriate manner.
17. Discuss the case regularly and collaborate effectively with the nonmedical therapist.
18. Consult the primary care team about psychiatric and substance abuse comorbidity with serious physical illness.
19. Learn the operation of various new technologies such as telepsychiatry.

Attitudes

At the end of training, the psychiatry resident should demonstrate understanding and knowledge of the following:

1. Empathy, respect, a nonjudgmental and collaborative approach, and the ability to tolerate ambiguity and display confidence in the efficacy of combined psychopharmacology and psychotherapy.
2. Sensitivity to the sociocultural, socioeconomic, and educational issues that arise within the therapeutic relationship.
3. The ability to establish an honest and receptive educational alliance with the supervisor and incorporate material discussed in supervision into psychotherapy.
4. The understanding that the individual components of integrated and split/collaborative treatment constitute the whole treatment and are not divisible into independent parts.
5. The ability to recognize obstacles to change and the ability to understand possible ways of addressing them.

6. An ethical commitment to put the patient's needs before one's own (Gabbard 2017).
7. Acceptance of possible audio recording, videotaping, or direct observation of treatment sessions.
8. Development of a positive alliance with the primary care team to treat patients with comorbid serious physical and mental illnesses.

Evaluation and Assessment Tool

As of this writing, no uniform evaluation tool is available to assess competencies across the field of psychiatry. Individual programs have tended to create assessment tools that are attuned to their training environment. We recommend that an evaluation tool or form be based on the three domains (knowledge, skills, and attitudes) to reflect residents' progress in the development of competency. For instance, the form could reflect whether a specific knowledge, skill, or attitude is a) not apparent, b) emerging, c) apparent, or d) well developed. An evaluation form could be a composite that serves as a summary of several cases (see "Requirements and Optimal Experience" below) or could be applied for each specific case and used for competency training and evaluation.

We also recommend establishing a log of supervisory times and patient contacts related to integrated and split/collaborative care activities. We found it useful and preferable for the competency supervisor to keep both the log of supervisory and patient contacts and the evaluation form (see "Requirements and Optimal Experience" below).

The evaluation form should serve as guidance during supervision of competency cases. Each program should also decide on the frequency of competency evaluations for combined (integrated or split/collaborative) pharmacotherapy and psychotherapy (e.g., every 3 months or at the termination of a particular case, depending on whether a composite or a case-specific form is used).

Other tools that could be used for the evaluation of combined pharmacotherapy and psychotherapy include video and/or audio recordings, direct observation, presentations at case conferences, and write-ups. One interesting research tool (Lopiccolo et al. 2005) looks at the degree of coordination as perceived by patients and clinicians involved in a clinical case. This tool may have value as an educational assessment.

Requirements and Optimal Experience

In designing outpatient supervision activities, psychiatric educators must consider a number of issues such as learning needs, patient population characteristics, and financial factors that may impinge on the training environment (Reardon et al. 2014). The optimal number of supervised and properly evaluated combined (integrated or split/collaborative) pharmacotherapy and psychotherapy competency cases is difficult to establish and depends on several factors, such as the availability of suitable patients and program caseload requirements for other psychotherapy competencies. The resident should preferably complete a minimum of six supervised and properly evaluated combined pharmacotherapy and psychotherapy cases during residency training. A minimum of three cases of integrated treatment and three cases of split/collaborative treatment should preferably be completed during adult psychiatry training.

Exposure to cases of combined pharmacotherapy and psychotherapy should start fairly early during training, in some cases during the second year of training (e.g., during consultation/liaison rotation or at the continuity clinic). The early start of competency training is especially pertinent for residents who plan to enter child and adolescent subspecialty training because they may have to finish all aspects of their adult psychiatry training by the end of the third year of training. Optimally, combined cases could be spread through the second, third, and fourth years.

There is no optimal or best setting for treating patients using the combination of pharmacotherapy and psychotherapy. Training in this treatment modality can occur with both inpatients and outpatients. However, the outpatient year of residency training may provide the most suitable opportunity because during this year the combined treatment could be executed in its entirety.

There are no specific selection criteria for selecting patients for combined pharmacotherapy and psychotherapy treatment. Each patient should receive an individual evaluation to determine whether a combination of pharmacotherapy and specific psychotherapy is suitable. Residents should consult with a clinical supervisor during the selection process. This said, we suggest caution regarding the selection of patients with very severe illness in the context of an acute episode (e.g., an acute exacerbation of psychosis or acute mania) as training cases for competency in combined pharmacotherapy and psychotherapy.

Supervision: Who, When, and How

Clinical supervision is accepted as a crucial part of clinical teaching (Farnan et al. 2012) and the formation of a capable clinical psychiatrist. Clinical supervision is valued "not only for training new practitioners, but also to ameliorate or prevent some of the adverse impact" of work as a mental health professional, and yet "there is limited research to support the claims that supervision actually has a positive impact on therapist well-being or leads to improved therapist practice and improved client outcomes" (Schofield and Grant 2013, p. 7). As a consequence, much of what we accept about clinical supervision relates to pedagogical traditions and anecdotal experience. We acknowledge these limitations as we seek to offer guidance on who, when, and how to conduct clinical supervision.

Given the absence of adequate data, the following question arises: What is proper supervision, proper monitoring, and a proper means of evaluation? The Royal College of Psychiatrists requirements call for at least 2 hours of individual supervision each week. However, the requirements for competency in three core areas of various psychotherapies and for competency in combined pharmacotherapy–psychotherapy treatment may actually press for more supervisory time. We advocate the use of separate expert supervisors for each competency (see below in this section). It may require a lot of juggling on the part of the resident to fit four supervisions into 2 hours, if the program adheres to having just 2 hours of supervision. Many residency programs provide for more supervision, frequently outside regular hours. However, even the extra supervision, together with the regular supervision, may still not provide enough time for all therapies and clinical issues every week. Residents and supervisors might decide not to meet for supervision for each specific psychotherapy (cognitive-behavioral therapy, psychodynamic therapy, etc.) every week, and the supervision of combined cases may become part of other psychotherapies supervision. Residents and supervisors may arrange supervision for some modalities one week and for other modalities on an alternate week. There might not be a need for supervision in some psychotherapies all the time (Schofield and Grant 2013); for instance, a resident may fulfill the requirements for brief psychotherapy (e.g., two completed cases) and therefore need no further supervision specifically focused on brief psychotherapy. However, the supervision should occur fairly regularly and frequently.

We recommend that programs delegate specific supervisors with some expertise in each particular psychotherapy competency if the staffing level is sufficient to do so. This does not mean that one supervisor could not or should not be a supervisor in more than one competency if he or she has some expertise in both (e.g., brief psychotherapy and psychodynamic psychotherapy). In cases in which one supervisor oversees more than one competency, specific supervision time should be devoted to each competency; the supervision of different competencies should not be lumped together.

Individuals who are assigned to supervise or oversee competency in combined (integrated or split/collaborative) pharmacotherapy and psychotherapy should be seasoned, clinically oriented psychiatrists who are well versed in pharmacotherapy, at least one psychotherapy modality, and the combination and also in supervising and collaborating with other mental health professionals. Graduate medical education regulations also require that residents are able to work effectively as members or leaders of a health care team and are able to act in a consultative role to other physicians and health professionals. Supervisors should keep in mind that becoming competent does not mean becoming an expert.

Proper individual supervision should address all three domains (knowledge, skills, and attitudes) of the combined pharmacotherapy and psychotherapy competency. As Gabbard (2017) points out, there are different means of evaluating competency (e.g., case write-ups, oral presentations at case conferences, written examinations, oral examinations, videotapes or direct observations, audiotape recordings, and individual supervision). The supervisor may select one or any combination of these for evaluating the resident. As Gabbard (2017) emphasizes, these methods of assessment all have certain advantages and disadvantages. Direct individual supervision over the course of training still seems the most useful in broadly evaluating all three competency domains.

Other means of evaluation, such as reviewing patients' charts, observing clinical interviews conducted by residents, and 360-degree evaluations (evaluation completed by several people [e.g., supervisors, collaborating nonmedical therapists, patients, patient families, colleagues, subordinates]), may be included to evaluate residents' competency.

Using a form developed on the basis of competency standards and domains reflecting the progress of acquiring competency may be helpful in supervision sessions. Progress in addressing deficiencies could be effectively monitored and documented by the use of such a form.

A special area of supervision and evaluation in split/collaborative treatment is the evaluation and supervision of collaboration with nonmedical therapists. Supervisors should monitor and address the content of communications between the resident and the nonmedical therapist. These communications should be regular and should not address crises only. Clashes and territory fights among professionals should be avoided and should be properly addressed in supervision when they do occur. Residents should properly collaborate with nonmedical therapists and should be able to discuss difficult situations with their collaborators. Residents should discuss each difficult interaction with a nonmedical therapist during their supervision and should seek the supervisor's advice. Supervisors should avoid addressing conflicts between residents and nonmedical therapists without consulting and having supervisors of the nonmedical therapists involved or present. The same applies to seasoned nonmedical therapists and supervisors of nonmedical therapists. In the rare case of a serious conflict, a meeting between the resident, the resident's supervisor, the nonmedical therapist, and the therapist's supervisor should be arranged to address and resolve the conflict.

Conclusion

Evaluation of competency in combined (either integrated or split/collaborative) pharmacotherapy and psychotherapy is a critical part of developing a proper level of competency as a psychiatrist. It is a complicated task that requires adequate time, supervisory expertise, and the development of specific evaluation tools. Supervisors may decide to use one or more evaluation tools such as an evaluation form, a log of contacts, direct observation, oral or written examination, and case presentations at conferences. Proper evaluation should address all aspects, standards, and domains of competency—namely, knowledge, skills, and attitudes. Special attention should be paid to the development of skills regarding how to collaborate with colleagues from across the health professions in the service of improved health care for patients in need.

References

Farnan JM, Petty LA, Georgitis E, et al: A systematic review: the effect of clinical supervision on patient and residency education outcomes. Acad Med 87(4):428–442, 2012 22361801

Gabbard GO: Long-Term Psychodynamic Psychotherapy: A Basic Text (Core Competencies in Psychotherapy Series), 3rd Edition. Arlington, VA, American Psychiatric Association Publishing, 2017

Guerrero APS, Beresin EV, Balon R, et al: The competency movement in psychiatric education. Acad Psychiatry 41(3):312–314, 2017 28382588

Lopiccolo CJ, Eldon Taylor C, Clemence C, et al: Split treatment: a measurement of coordination between psychiatrists. Psychiatry (Edgmont) 2(1):43–46, 2005 21179642

Merriam-Webster: Merriam-Webster's Collegiate Dictionary, 11th Edition. Springfield, MA, Merriam-Webster, 2003

Reardon C, May M, Williams K: Psychiatry resident outpatient clinic supervision: how training directors are balancing patient care, education, and reimbursement. Acad Psychiatry 38(4):476–480, 2014 24664608

Sargent J, Mohl PC, Beitman BB, et al: Psychotherapy Combined With Psychopharmacology Competencies. Farmington, CT, American Association of Directors of Psychiatry Residency Training, 2001. Available at: http://www. aadprt.org/public/ educators.html. Accessed December 1, 2004

Scheiber SC, Kramer TAM: What core competencies mean to psychiatrists and trainees, in Core Competencies for Psychiatric Practice: What Clinicians Need to Know: A Report of the American Board of Psychiatry and Neurology. Edited by Scheiber SC, Kramer TAM, Adamowski SE. Washington, DC, American Psychiatric Publishing, 2003, pp 3–5

Schofield MJ, Grant J: Developing psychotherapists' competence through clinical supervision: protocol for a qualitative study of supervisory dyads. BMC Psychiatry 13(12), 2013 23298408

Termination in
Integrated and
Split/Collaborative
Treatment

9

Integrated or split/collaborative treatment may continue indefinitely in some cases of serious or recurrent major mental disorder. In many cases, however, integrated and split/collaborative treatment may transition or be terminated by the preference or circumstances of the patient or the recommendation of the psychiatrist. Termination in either model of treatment could mean either simultaneous termination of pharmacotherapy and psychotherapy (although this is rarely done) or sequenced termination, with either pharmacotherapy or psychotherapy being transitioned first and the other modality being terminated later.

The simultaneous termination of both modalities may be precipitated by the patient, either by requesting it and discussing it with the treating psychiatrist or simply by not showing up for treatment. As Bender and Messner (2003) point out, these patients are not formally "terminating" their care but are essentially opting out of treatment. Patients may feel that they have improved sufficiently or that the benefits of continued therapy have been significantly diminishing

(Makover 2016). Another rather unfortunate and perhaps the most frequent reason for termination of treatment is the patient's lack of resources to continue; either the third-party payer decides that the cost is too great (Makover 2016) or covers only a predetermined number of sessions per specific disorder or condition, or the patient, paying out of pocket for treatment, runs out of money.

A special case of termination occurs during residency training: many patients treated by residents are transferred to another resident after the treating resident moves to a new phase of the curriculum or leaves the program. Although this is not a true *treatment* termination, it is a termination of a therapeutic relationship, and as such it also needs to be carefully planned and executed. Finally, the decision to refer the patient for psychotherapy after an initial period of pharmacotherapy (medication management) while pharmacotherapy continues (split/collaborative arrangement) may be viewed by the patient as termination and should be handled in a similar fashion in some cases.

Termination of any treatment should always be planned well ahead, preferably several months in advance. Makover (2016) even suggests that the planning for termination should begin at the start of treatment. The sequencing of termination is a complicated process that depends on various factors, including the diagnosis; severity of illness; efficacy and outcome of integrated treatment so far; psychotherapeutic modality used; overall treatment goals; treatment goals of each modality; the patient's preferences, beliefs, and misconceptions; medication side effects; and, unfortunately, financial resources.

The case of major depression provides an example of the complexity of termination sequencing in integrated or split/collaborative treatment. For a patient with a single episode of major depression, the resident may consider terminating the course of cognitive-behavioral therapy after 12 sessions and significant improvement but continuing antidepressant treatment for another several months to achieve the recommended 6- to 9-month period of stable improvement. In another case of a single episode of major depression, the resident may consider terminating antidepressant treatment after 9 months of stable improvement while continuing cognitive-behavioral therapy or supportive psychotherapy, for example, to address adjustment to a new job or marital problems. In the case of recurrent major depression, the resident may terminate psychotherapy and continue antidepressant treatment indefinitely. With treatment-resistant major depression, the patient may undergo a series of treatments with repetitive transcranial magnetic stimulation or electroconvulsive therapy, plus ongoing medication and psychotherapy, in order for symptoms to be adequately addressed.

Moreover, with termination of care, transitioning from multiple therapeutic modalities and clinicians may be involved. Recommendations on the sequencing of biological and psychosocial intervention transitions vary, but some (e.g., Fava and Ruini 2002; Fava and Visani 2008) advocate for sequencing pharmacotherapy and presumably circuit-based interventions first, followed by psychotherapy. This approach is thought to create a greater psychosocial "safety net" and may have advantages in preventing relapse.

Giving greater attention to the remaining therapeutic intervention is advantageous. Providing more intensive psychotherapy, for example, could be extremely helpful during the period in which medication treatment is being transitioned. Such efforts could help lessen some of the patient's anxieties about stopping medication.

The resident should be aware that termination of either pharmacotherapy or psychotherapy can be very difficult and may trigger strong transferential and countertransferential responses. Ideally, termination of treatment occurs through careful, mutual treatment planning decisions and is the result of a true collaborative alliance between the clinician and patient. During psychiatric training, a resident may at times be forced to terminate one or both treatment modalities unilaterally (e.g., graduating from the program or because of the patient's lack of adherence to treatment, continuous substance abuse, or failure to pay for treatment). Such terminations may be challenging for patients and residents alike, and a poor process in transferring clinical care from one provider to another may introduce risk for certain psychiatrically fragile patients (Young and Eisendrath 2011). Recommendations for residents who transfer patients to others include the following: preparing patients for the transition, using digital platforms to communicate essential information, balancing caseloads so that new clinicians are not overwhelmed when accepting a transferred patient, identifying and protecting high-risk patients, increasing supervision and monitoring of residents during the time of transition, requiring explicit written and verbal handoffs, maintaining phone contact with the patient during the initial week of the transition, and requiring collaboration with other members of the clinical care team.

For more established psychiatrists in clinical practice, similar steps should be undertaken. Gabbard (2017, p. 197) points out that "[i]n most states, it is perfectly legal to discontinue treatment with a patient provided that suicidality or danger to others has been carefully assessed" and appropriate follow-up has been arranged. He suggests that psychiatrists should provide the notice of termination in writing and list potential care providers in case the patient would like to seek treatment in the future.

At the time of formal termination of care, the clinician should provide "reasonable notice," which is an appropriate period of time for the patient to adjust to the decision and explore any concerns. The clinician should offer education, future treatment recommendations, and guidance about when and/or where to seek care in the future, should it be needed. A thorough discussion of potential resources should occur, and the clinician should document the reasons for termination. A follow-up letter to the patient with information about the condition, the type of treatment that was provided, and future care options may also be a valuable practice in most settings (Young and Eisendrath 2011; Young et al. 2011).

The decision about sequencing the termination of pharmacotherapy and psychotherapy in integrated treatment is *relatively* easier than in collaborative or split treatment, because it involves fewer individuals.

Competency

Psychiatry residents should be able to demonstrate the factors that are helpful in terminating care with patients.

Terminating Pharmacotherapy First

The discussion about terminating pharmacotherapy frequently starts at the beginning of medication treatment. This discussion is frequently triggered by the patient's uneasiness about taking psychotropic medication. Besides asking about the side effects, one of the first questions many patients ask is, "How long will I have to take these pills?" An honest answer, including the possibility that the psychiatrist does not know or is not sure, should follow.

The initial discussion of treatment and formulation of the treatment plan should always include the goals of each treatment modality and the possible best time for the termination of each treatment type (Beitman et al. 2003). This discussion should be specific (to the extent possible) and clear. For instance, specifying the duration of pharmacotherapy in the case of the first episode of major depression is relatively easy. The patient should know that he or she will continue taking the antidepressant (at its full dosage) for 6–9 months after reaching remission, which in lay terms means after starting to feel and function well. The issue of counting the duration of the continuation of pharmacotherapy from the time of feeling well is important. It can frequently take 2–3 months to reach full remission. Patients may start to press for termination of medication in another 3 months—clearly an insufficient amount of time.

The suggested length of pharmacotherapy varies from disorder to disorder and depends on various factors (e.g., chronicity, severity, and recurrence of the disorder; previous response and adherence to medication; family history; presence of stresses). In many cases, the discontinuation of medication is not a simple process accomplished by merely saying, "No more pills starting tomorrow." Many psychotropic medications need to be discontinued gradually, some over a period of a few days and some over a period of a few weeks (e.g., high dosages of alprazolam). Even some antidepressants—for example, venlafaxine or paroxetine—may be quite difficult to discontinue because of discontinuation or withdrawal symptoms. Because polypharmacy has become quite common, discontinuation of medications can become quite a complicated task. An example would be a patient treated with an antidepressant, a mood stabilizer, and a hypnotic. Which one should be stopped first? Second? We suggest that the resident never discontinue more than one medication at the same time. The sequencing of the discontinuation of several medications should be individualized, and all the general suggestions about discontinuation should be applied to each particular medication.

The initial planning of pharmacotherapy termination should also include the discussion of what will happen with psychotherapy. The patient should clearly understand that terminating pharmacotherapy *does not* inevitably mean terminating psychotherapy. Finally, the initial discussion may include the issues of recurrence of symptoms and follow-up after pharmacotherapy termination. However, these issues may come up more frequently during the process of termination itself.

Beitman et al. (2003) and others suggest that in longer-term psychotherapy, it is best to announce anticipated termination early in the process, at least 3–6 months ahead of time. Mischoulon and colleagues (2000) also suggest the general timeline of 3–6 months for announcing termination. They also provide several suggestions for ameliorating a change in psychopharmacologist, which may be adapted for termination of pharmacotherapy.

These modified suggestions include informing the patient that symptoms may worsen transiently after the termination, reminding the patient of termination during each visit in the termination phase, allowing the patient to verbalize his or her feelings, and even using a standardized protocol for transfer and termination (Mischoulon et al. 2000).

We believe that the discussion of medication termination should also include additional clinical issues such as the following:

1. The possibility of physiological as well as psychological withdrawal symptoms after stopping the medication (not only with benzodiazepines but also with some selective serotonin reuptake inhibitors, serotonin norepinephrine reuptake inhibitors, and other psychotropic medications). Discussion should include the timeline of these symptoms (e.g., withdrawal symptoms after the discontinuation of some benzodiazepines with long half-lives may be delayed for 1–2 weeks, whereas withdrawal symptoms associated with alprazolam may occur almost immediately) and a plan for their management.
2. The chance of increased suicidality during the discontinuation phase of some medications, particularly after the discontinuation of lithium (e.g., Lewitzka et al. 2015).
3. Aftercare monitoring of withdrawal symptoms, recurrence symptoms, suicidality, and other clinical issues (which, in the case of continuing psychotherapy, should not be difficult). In case any unusual symptoms occur, patients

should be encouraged to contact the resident as soon as possible and at any time. Use of digital diaries or electronic health apps to track symptoms may be advisable.

4. Avoidance of triggers of various symptoms. This means maintaining a healthy lifestyle, including avoiding or limiting the use of alcohol, caffeine, and tobacco; exercising; and getting regular and sufficient sleep.

5. Reassurance to the patient that the issues of medication discontinuation can be freely discussed during several subsequent psychotherapy sessions. However, the issue of medication discontinuation should not become a dominating concern in continuing psychotherapy.

Residents should always discuss the termination plan with their clinical and psychotherapy supervisors.

Competency

Psychiatry residents should be able to demonstrate the skills and knowledge to terminate pharmacotherapy with a patient when both pharmacotherapy and psychotherapy were provided by the resident.

Terminating Psychotherapy First

Termination of psychotherapy in integrated treatment while pharmacotherapy continues is usually a more complicated task than terminating pharmacotherapy first. Psychotherapy may be terminated, as mutually agreed, after certain goals of psychotherapy have been achieved (probably more frequently in a course of cognitive-behavioral therapy, brief psychotherapy, or supportive psychotherapy than in long-term psychodynamic psychotherapy). Termination of psychotherapy in integrated treatment specifically may also be forced by various circumstances, such as 1) the patient or therapist feeling that there is no value in continuing psychotherapy; 2) relocation of either the patient or the physician, including graduation and change of rotation of the resident (this also forces simultaneous termination of pharmacotherapy); or 3) economic reasons (either the third-party payer refuses to pay for more sessions, the patient paying out of pocket runs out of money, or the number of sessions was predetermined from the beginning).

Similar to pharmacotherapy, the initial discussion of treatment and formulation of the treatment plan should always include the goals of psychotherapy and the best possible time for termination (Beitman et al. 2003). The time frame of psychotherapy termination should always be individualized. The fact that the timing of termination may be predetermined (a number of sessions agreed on from the beginning or forced by the third-party payer) does not necessarily make the termination easier and does not mean that termination should not be carefully planned and executed. Termination should be discussed for several sessions before the last psychotherapy session. Ideally, the resident would allow for a time frame similar to the 3–6 months in the case of pharmacotherapy. However, some psychotherapy modalities (cognitive-behavioral therapy and brief psychotherapy) have shorter durations and thus do not allow for such a long termination process. It is generally recommended that the patient should be informed about the planned date of termination at the beginning of psychotherapy in cases of forced termination with a known termination date (e.g., the resident knows that he or she will be leaving the service or training program in a year).

The patient's readiness for termination should be regularly assessed during the termination phase of psychotherapy. The termination process frequently brings up a number of transference issues. "Some patients may start flooding each remaining session with a barrage of new material, pushing themselves to discuss previously avoided material" (Bender and Messner 2003, p. 297). The patient may become openly hostile or angry, may miss sessions or come late, and may regress or even decompensate (Bender and Messner 2003). Many training programs witness an increase of regressing or decompensated patients, who continue taking medications, during the May–June period when residents terminate their long-term cases before departing from residency. A special issue in integrated treatment may be the threat of noncompliance or lack of adherence with pharmacotherapy regimens. It is well known that psychotherapy induces stronger compliance with pharmacotherapy with the combination of treatment modalities (e.g., in depression; see Pampallona et al. 2004). When psychotherapy is being terminated but the treatment plan calls for continuing medication for various reasons (mainly the prevention of relapse or attenuation of residual symptoms), the patient may threaten to skip or stop taking the medication. The dangers of terminating medication—especially terminating suddenly—need to be included in the discussion of termination. However, the continuation of pharmacotherapy (we are discussing terminating psychotherapy while pharmacotherapy is continuing) could provide some help in terminating psychotherapy, as the doctor–patient relationship will continue. Pharmacotherapy sessions may be used for some therapeutic support, for prevention of decompensation, or for addressing the decompensation after the termination of psychotherapy.

The process of termination may also give rise to various countertransference issues. These issues may interfere with a careful assessment of the patient's readiness to terminate psychotherapy. Gabbard (2017) points out several countertransference issues that could play a role in planning and executing psychotherapy termination by any therapist, including residents. Residents may overestimate or idealize psychotherapy and avoid conducting a proper, well-planned termination. Residents may also hold on to patients for their own emotional needs. Certain patients may enhance the resident's self-esteem, making the termination difficult if not impossible. However, countertransference may also force premature termination, because some patients may arouse deep feelings of loss and negative emotions such as boredom and anger in residents (Gabbard 2017; Schen et al. 2013). The resident should always discuss these termination issues with their supervisor (Roberts 2016).

Termination of psychotherapy may also lead to an increase in the permeability of boundaries (Gabbard 2017). Patients may be inclined to ask more personal questions and might offer gifts or hugs. However, such issues might not arise as frequently when terminating psychotherapy in integrated treatment while pharmacotherapy continues. Nevertheless, residents should be aware of the possibility of these boundary issues. Should gifts be accepted as a well-meant symbol of termination, or should they be rejected and discussed? Should a hug be accepted or rejected? What about suggestions of future meetings outside of the office after psychotherapy termination? These are complicated issues that need to be addressed on an individual basis and in a frame of proper supervision (Roberts 2016).

We recommend that the termination of psychotherapy be well planned in advance and structured according to the following guidelines:

1. Termination of psychotherapy is announced and planned either from the very beginning in the case of time-limited therapies or several months in advance in the case of long-term psychotherapy.
2. The patient's feelings, worries, transference, and reaction to psychotherapy termination are regularly explored, discussed, and addressed. The patient should be actively invited to verbalize his or her feelings about termination during several termination sessions.
3. In some cases, the patient could be offered several intermittent, as-needed termination sessions between pharmacotherapy appointments. Psychotherapy may be tapered off this way (e.g., from once a week to once a month to occasionally none) while pharmacotherapy continues. Future "booster" sessions may be offered on an individual basis.
4. Possible decompensation, acting out, recurrence of symptoms, and occurrence of suicidality should be carefully monitored.
5. Medication adjustments or addition may occasionally be offered to manage various symptoms or decompensation during termination.
6. Increased attention to adherence to the originally prescribed medication regimen (i.e., continuing pharmacotherapy) is recommended.
7. The patient should be reassured that the doctor–patient relationship is not terminated and that some therapeutic issues can be brought up during the course of continuing pharmacotherapy. The resident should be careful,

however, that this does not sabotage the entire process of termination and that the patient does not surreptitiously bring the therapy back. Junior residents have a tendency to continue full-fledged psychotherapy during medication review appointments.

8. Just as during termination of pharmacotherapy, patients should be educated that avoiding stressors such as emotional conflicts could be helpful during termination of psychotherapy.
9. The resident should be aware of the increased possibility of boundary violations during termination of psychotherapy.
10. The resident should always seek proper and frequent supervision to address all termination issues.

Competency

Psychiatry residents should be able to demonstrate the skills and knowledge to terminate psychotherapy with a patient when both pharmacotherapy and psychotherapy were provided by the resident.

A final word about termination: Contrary to previously held views, termination does not necessarily mean a permanent ending. Bender and Messner (2003) point out that "while it is important to view a therapy's termination as a completion of a piece of work, this does not mean that future (professional) meetings cannot occur" (p. 306). Many psychiatrists and therapists explicitly invite their patients to call them in the future, for example, in cases of setbacks or relapse.

Terminating Pharmacotherapy and Psychotherapy at the Same Time

Simultaneous termination of pharmacotherapy and psychotherapy in integrated treatment in everyday practice is usually rare. However, simultaneous termination of both pharmacotherapy and psychotherapy occurs fairly frequently in residency training programs at the time when residents terminate their cases before graduating or changing services. Usually, this is not a true termination of treatment or treatment modality as discussed in this chapter so far, but a termination of the doctor–patient relationship and transfer to another resident. This process can be quite demanding and difficult.

Simultaneous termination stirs up similar feelings as those that occur during termination of psychotherapy or pharmacotherapy separately. Patients may feel angry, devastated, and abandoned. For some patients, this is a déjà vu experience they go through several times while being treated in training programs.

Transfer to another resident should be carefully planned, and the planning should start several (3–6) months in advance. The plan should include all issues about termination of psychotherapy discussed in this chapter. In addition, it may be helpful to arrange an early meeting with the new resident (Mischoulon et al. 2000). The departing resident may emphasize the benefits of a new physician, including a fresh outlook and new ideas (Mischoulon et al. 2000). The departing resident may also offer a few scheduled telephone sessions during this period of transition (Bender and Messner 2003) and offer to be available over the telephone or by e-mail in case of a crisis. However, the boundaries and rules of these contacts should be set at the beginning of treatment. We have also found the use of support staff helpful in the process of transition. A good, empathic support staff could provide a symbol of permanence in contrast to the yearly changing residents and may help to smooth the transition.

The rules of transfer apply not only to transfers within the residency training program but also to any mutually agreeable and planned transfer of the patient in clinical practice. The departing (because of retirement, relocation, illness, or another reason) psychiatrist should provide the patient with a referral and then should apply rules similar to those discussed for transfer within the residency training program. These recommendations similarly apply to termination due to patient relocation.

The simultaneous termination of pharmacotherapy and psychotherapy requires combining the recommendations for termination of pharmacotherapy and psychotherapy. We do not recommend actually terminating both simultaneously, however, because of a number of possible complications and difficulties associated with this process. Instead, we recommend sequencing the termination of integrated treatment, starting with either pharmacotherapy or psychotherapy. As pointed out, sequencing should be individualized and should depend on numerous clinical, personal, and economic factors.

Transfer to another therapist or true simultaneous termination also requires addressing posttermination psychiatrist–patient boundary issues (Malmquist and Notman 2001; Schen et al. 2013). The posttermination time is a period of increased probability and propensity for boundary violations, which can range from accepting improper gifts to emotional or sexual involvement. The discussion of proper posttreatment boundaries (the same boundaries that exist during treatment) should always be included in termination planning.

It is extremely important not to abandon the patient during the process of termination. *Patient abandonment* means the unilateral termination of care without sufficient notice and without adequate planning around an alternative resource for care if necessary. Moreover, termination—and abandonment—may be viewed differently from the perspective of the patient than from that of the clinician. For these reasons, it is especially important to approach the process carefully and with mutual dialogue and decision making. A wise clinician will document the process well and will provide a letter to the patient outlining the issues discussed as well as future clinical care options.

Competency

Psychiatry residents should be able to demonstrate the skills and knowledge to terminate both pharmacotherapy and psychotherapy with a patient when both pharmacotherapy and psychotherapy were provided by the resident.

Termination is an important part of any therapeutic process; its proper planning and implementation must be an essential part of competent treatment. Termination should also lay the groundwork for enhanced self-care, monitoring, and health practices of the patient and should lessen barriers to care, should it be necessary in the future.

References

Beitman BD, Blinder BJ, Thase ME, et al: Integrating Psychotherapy and Pharmacotherapy: Dissolving the Mind-Brain Barrier. New York, WW Norton 2003

Bender S, Messner E: Becoming a Therapist: What Do I Say, and Why? New York, Guilford, 2003

Fava GA, Ruini C: The sequential approach to relapse prevention in unipolar depression. World Psychiatry 1(1):10–15, 2002 16946806

Fava GA, Visani D: Psychosocial determinants of recovery in depression. Dialogues Clin Neurosci 10(4):461–472, 2008 19170403

Gabbard GO: Long-Term Psychodynamic Psychotherapy: A Basic Text, 3rd Edition (Core Competencies in Psychotherapy Series). Arlington, VA, American Psychiatric Association Publishing, 2017

Lewitzka U, Severus E, Bauer R, et al: The suicide prevention effect of lithium: more than 20 years of evidence—a narrative review. Int J Bipolar Disord 3(1):32, 2015 26183461

Makover RB: Treatment Planning for Psychotherapists: A Practical Guide to Better Outcomes, 3rd Edition. Arlington, VA, American Psychiatric Publishing, 2016

Malmquist CP, Notman MT: Psychiatrist-patient boundary issues following treatment termination. Am J Psychiatry 158(7):1010–1018, 2001 11431220

Mischoulon D, Rosenbaum JF, Messner E: Transfer to a new psychopharmacologist: its effect on patients. Acad Psychiatry 24:156–163, 2000

Pampallona S, Bollini P, Tibaldi G, et al: Combined pharmacotherapy and psychological treatment for depression: a systematic review. Arch Gen Psychiatry 61(7):714–719, 2004 15237083

Roberts LW: A Clinical Guide to Psychiatric Ethics. Arlington, VA, American Psychiatric Association Publishing, 2016

Schen CR, Raymond L, Notman M: Transfer of care of psychotherapy patients: implications for psychiatry training. Psychodyn Psychiatry 41(4):575–595, 2013 24283450

Young JQ, Eisendrath SJ: Enhancing patient safety and resident education during the academic year-end transfer of outpatients: lessons from the suicide of a psychiatric patient. Acad Psychiatry 35(1):54–57, 2011 21209409

Young JQ, Pringle Z, Wachter RM: Improving follow-up of high-risk psychiatry outpatients at resident year-end transfer. Jt Comm J Qual Patient Saf 37(7):300–308, 2011 21819028

Primary Care and Split/Collaborative Care

10

Improving Access, Decreasing Costs, Improving Outcomes

The need to better address mental health in the primary care setting emerged over 30 years ago, with the realization that primary care physicians in the United States treat the majority of patients with mental health problems (Katon et al. 2010b). Primary care physicians are responsible for most psychotropic prescriptions, and as early as 2001, physicians in primary care settings wrote twice the number of prescriptions for antidepressant medication as psychiatrists (Voelker 2001). In 2014, approximately 18% of adults in the United States experienced some form of mental health disorder, and 8% had a substance use disorder (Knickman et al. 2016). Most individuals in need of treatment receive care in primary care settings rather than in psychiatrists' or psychologists' offices. Moreover, mental health and substance abuse disorders are often accompanied by comorbidities, such as cardiovascular disease and diabetes. A recent review performed by the Academy of Psychosomatic Medicine identified more than 600 articles in the literature that substantiate the finding that integrated and collaborative care strategies "have been consistently successful in improving key outcomes in both research and clinical intervention studies; cost analyses also suggest that this model is cost-effective" (Huffman et al. 2014, p. 109.

Indeed, co-occurring disorders appear to be the rule rather than the exception, and beyond their emotional cost, the economic burden that they generate is staggering. The additional costs associated with co-occurring mental and physical health issues or comorbidities have been estimated to reach $293 billion each year in the United States (Melek et al. 2014). More positively, the net savings that could be achieved through intentional efforts to integrate physical and mental health care in primary care settings has been determined to range from $26.3 to $48.3 billion annually (Melek et al. 2014).

Given these complex issues, it is likely that most patients with co-occurring psychiatric and other chronic medical conditions will be under the care of more than one clinician. In the primary care setting, the primary care physician is usually the prescriber, although the prescriber might also be a psychiatrist or nurse practitioner or other type of physician, such as a specialist (e.g., cardiologist, oncologist). The therapist could be a social worker, family therapist, psychologist, nurse practitioner, school counselor—or a psychiatrist. In a large study by Wiles and colleagues (2013) in the United Kingdom, for example, cognitive-behavioral therapy delivered by therapists with a variety of professional backgrounds was found to be effective as an adjunct to pharmacotherapy, prescribed by general practitioners, for patients with treatment-resistant depression.

Many factors have led to the increase in split/collaborative treatment over the last 30 years, including a wider variety of effective and safe medications for anxiety, depression, and psychosis; increased numbers of social workers, psychologists, and nurse practitioners; decreased stigma regarding receiving care for psychiatric problems; identification of patients with mental illness at earlier ages, including during childhood and adolescence; increased screening and awareness of psychiatric problems in primary care; and direct-to-consumer advertising by pharmaceutical companies on television, radio, and in print media (Riba 2001).

Yet, systems of care for the evaluation and treatment of general medical, mental health, and substance use disorders are not cohesive or well coordinated. As elegantly reviewed by Knickman et al. (2016), three key system-level barriers impede more effective care:

- Health care in the United States is highly fragmented, with separate, unintegrated medical care systems, mental health care systems, substance use service systems, and insurance networks, as well as often-needed social service systems.

- The workforce serving patients with co-occurring psychiatric and medical conditions is undersized, poorly distributed, and underprepared for the challenges. There are not enough psychiatrists, psychologists, social workers, and substance use counselors, and there is a large regional variation in the availability of these professionals. Furthermore, these clinicians are not adequately trained to work in teams to deliver medical, social, and behavioral evidence-based services.
- Existing payment systems do not adequately incentivize or provide the required resources to deliver effective care.

As reviewed by Schwenk (2016), the realization of the need for mental health care providers to work more closely and in partnership with primary care providers has led to a progressive number of changes over the years, including adding mental health professionals to primary care offices; enhancing training of primary care clinicians regarding basic problem-focused psychotherapy; making psychiatrists and other mental health professionals available, either in person or by telepsychiatry, by phone, or other means to primary care clinicians; improving patient registries to allow the assessment and monitoring of mental health care; and establishing collaborative care models in large integrated health systems. Many of the early studies of these collaborative care models focused on improving the care of patients with chronic medical diseases—such as hypertension and diabetes—among patients with mental illness (Katon et al. 2010a).

In a recent retrospective study by Reiss-Brennan et al. (2016) comparing the association of receiving primary care in integrated team-based care practices with traditional practice management, exposure to team-based care was associated with significant and substantial reductions in emergency department visits, hospital admissions, and primary care visits but no difference in urgent care or specialty physician visits. For those patients with complex mental illness and chronic medical diseases, team-based care was found to be superior to traditional practice management (Reiss-Brennan et al. 2016). Small private medical practices face major challenges because they do not have the economies of scale that large systems have to absorb the staffing, training, and support and information technology that are needed for such collaborative care models (Schwenk 2016).

With new models of funding needed for such delivery, the Centers for Medicare & Medicaid Services has begun reimbursement for collaborative care services. Called the Collaborative Care Model (CoCM), the primary health care provider employs a behavioral health care manager to provide ongoing care management for a caseload of patients with diagnosed mental health or substance use disorders. The psychiatrist provides a primary care practice with expert advice and consultation through regular case review and recommendations for treatment and medication adjustments in the care of specific patients; in especially difficult cases, the psychiatrist may also provide direct treatment.

The Collaborative Care Model

In the CoCM model, the behavioral health provider or case manager receives patient information and additional data and makes contact with patients at regular intervals and then gives guidance to primary care clinicians regarding their patients' behavioral health problems. This approach allows for consultation and collaboration, which occur within days or weeks instead of months, thereby providing better access to care for individuals in need of services. For patients with more challenging problems, in-house visits in person can be arranged. The psychiatrist has regular (weekly) meetings with a behavioral health provider/care manager, reviews the cases of all patients who are not improving, and makes treatment recommendations. With this method, the psychiatrist provides input on 10–20 patients in a half day, as opposed to 3–4 patients. With multiple brief consultations, there is more opportunity to "correct the course" if patients are not improving (Ratzliff and Unützer 2016).

The principles of CoCM are based on evidence and are population based, measurement based, and patient centered. The collaborative care team is led by a primary care provider. The functions of the behavioral health provider, the care manager, and the psychiatric consultant are clearly delineated, in which the care manager supports the primary care provider and uses evidence-based tools, and the psychiatric consultant provides recommendations. The role of the psychiatric consultant in this model is to carry out the following:

- Review cases with the care manager using the registry.
- Prioritize patients who are not improving.
- Provide treatment recommendation to the primary care team.
- Consult urgently as needed.

Common consultation questions relate to the following:

- Clarifying the diagnosis
- Addressing treatment-resistant disorders
- Making recommendations for managing difficult patients

For patients who do not improve, for example, the consultant might consider if an incorrect diagnosis was made, if there are problems with treatment adherence, if the dose or duration of treatment is insufficient, or if side effects are occurring. The consultant might also consider other complicating factors such as psychosocial stressors, medical problems, substance abuse, and other psychiatric problems.

Another important aspect of collaborative care is the use of innovative technology. For example, psychiatrists may be available for evaluation or consultation via telepsychiatry. Mobile applications, such as smartphone apps, provide patients the opportunity to check in with their clinicians and care team members anytime. Such technology-based activities may afford a deeper partnership and development of the therapeutic alliance that might not be so easily formed without such devices. In addition, such technology allows for check-ins; improved medication adherence; and the ability to look at sleep, substance use, nutrition, exercise, and interaction with family and friends on a real-time basis. In addition, specific types of psychotherapy—such as basic problem-solving therapy or therapy based on cognitive-behavioral techniques—can be provided by smartphone apps or other Web-based technologies, opening up the door to improved access and more cost-effective and self-determined types of care. Special populations—such as returning veterans or employees who are working in other countries or remote locations—have been shown to be well served throughout different stages of care through the use of such developing technologies, as evidenced in several activities of the VAH mental health system in the United States.

There are, however, practical aspects of collaborative care that still need to be developed. Traditionally, mental health professionals and primary care physicians have treated patients concurrently, that is, "in parallel," rather than collaboratively (Valenstein 1999). When patients refer themselves for mental health care, the primary care physician might never be informed let alone collaborate with the mental health provider. In addition, the level and quality of communication from the mental health provider to the primary care provider have been viewed as less than ideal in a study by Brown and Weston (1992).

In the last 30 years, several collaborative care models have been proposed, piloted, and implemented, moving away from the traditional "parallel" patient treatment. In general, however, most collaborative treatments have been worked out by individual providers on a case-by-case basis. The large collaborative care studies, such as CoCM discussed above, are comprehensive, thoughtful, and well funded. For the individual practitioner, there remain a number of issues to ponder. For example, there are liability issues for psychiatrists who are not actually seeing and examining patients themselves but who are talking with care managers and behavioral health providers about management and treatment issues. To some extent, this harkens back to the days when psychiatrists were not comfortable seeing large numbers of patients in community mental health settings, where patients were seen mostly by social workers and psychologists, whereas psychiatrists were mostly being used to prescribe medications. The risk and liability issues with that model meant that many psychiatrists did not find it meaningful to prescribe medications without providing psychotherapy. A practical aspect for small private practitioners is that there is not an economy of scale to set up systems for care managers and behavioral providers. It takes a lot of time and effort to call primary care providers and wait for returned calls, to have electronic medical records that can "talk" with a number of primary care clinics, and to set up times for teams to collaborate and communicate about and with the patients. The practical aspects of this type of care are quite complex. Furthermore, it is essential to consider how best to train attending physicians and group and solo practitioners in collaborative care methodology—many are busy and already have routines and panels of patients.

Potential Pitfalls in Split/Collaborative Treatment With Primary Care Practitioners

Poor Communication

Even though we rely on medical records more and more, patients may not disclose, and we may not ask about, who else the patient is seeing for care. The patient may be embarrassed to admit that he or she is seeing a mental health professional or may not feel it is germane to the chronic medical condition. The primary care physician and mental health professional may not know each other and may therefore not find it useful to communicate. There may be a myriad of reasons and obstacles for poor communication. Gitlin and Miklowitz (2016) wrote about the low frequency of communication between psychopharmacologist and therapist, and it is plausible that the communication between the resident and primary care physician is not very frequent either, although good data on the issue do not exist. Communication between these two parties should occur when there is a change of diagnosis, a change in symptomatology, emergent suicidality, major side effects, and possibility of medication interactions. The primary care physician may be able to detect certain side effects better (e.g., QT prolongation, weight gain, changes in glycemia with atypical antipsychotics, increased blood pressure with venlafaxine). Residents and primary care physicians may discuss management of some side effects—for example, hypothyroidism associated with lithium, use of antihypertensives in cases of venlafaxine- or duloxetine-associated increase of blood pressure, augmentation of antidepressants with levothyroxine, or use of metformin in weight gain associated with atypical antipsychotics. On the initial contact between the resident or therapist and the primary care physician, it should be decided how the participating parties will communicate, whether by telephone, mail, or e-mail. Care providers should also be aware of the possibility of splitting by the patient and subsequent countertransference, not only toward the patient but also toward each other. Last but not least, as Gitlin and Miklowitz (2016) note, mutual respect in this communication is vital.

Overvaluation of Medication

Some patients, as well as clinicians, overvalue medication and view most psychiatric problems within the realm of a "chemical imbalance." Although psychotropic medications work well in many cases, they do not work well for everyone. They only work with the correct diagnosis, and they only work if there is proper adherence; for many conditions, there needs to be a combination of psychotherapy and pharmacotherapy to achieve optimal outcomes. If all these conditions are not met, the patient may think that the problem is with the specific medication, rather than with the host of factors that may be contributing (Riba 2001).

Roles of the Clinicians

Side effects of medications are very problematic. No party (i.e., primary care physician or resident), however, should change the medication prescribed by the other because of its side effects (unless the side effects are life-threatening). This should be discussed at the outset of collaboration. If these issues are not expressly discussed by defining the roles of the clinicians ahead of time (i.e., who is prescribing and monitoring medication), then there may be failures in treatment.

Role of Psychotherapy

In a busy clinical practice with a large panel of patients, primary care physicians may not be able to determine and appreciate the role of psychotherapy, and the specific type of psychotherapy that a particular patient might need. Similarly, if the therapist (in cases in which the primary care physician collaborates just with a therapist) undervalues the role of medication, this type of treatment might not be provided in a timely way. The role of psychotherapy may therefore either be overvalued or devalu15ed (Riba 2001).

Transference and Countertransference

Patients develop transference toward clinicians, and clinicians develop countertransference toward patients. When patients have more than one clinician, such as in a split/collaborative arrangement, factoring in the value of the work of one clinician versus another becomes complicated for the patient, especially if one clinician is providing psychotherapy and another is providing medications and other treatments. It is important for the primary care physician to realize that providing medication (psychotropic medication) requires an understanding of the psychology of prescribing—how to work to enable the patient to adhere to the medication, how certain factors might prove the treatment plan unsuccessful, how certain psychosocial or financial issues may play a role, and how the patient's feelings toward the primary care physician contribute to the efficacy of medication. The role and importance of medication and psychotherapy may shift for the patient as the treatment progresses and changes (Riba 2001).

General Issues for Training Residents

A widely acceptable training model is not available at the present time. The integrated care model is clearly in need of clinical consultants, clinical educators, and clinical team leaders (Ratzliff et al. 2015). As new models for effective care and partnership with primary care physicians continue to emerge, it is important for residents to think about the following:

1. Residents might want to seek training during residency that will give them an opportunity to have didactic and clinical experiences working with primary care clinicians, preferably in various treatment settings. Such experiences might include electives with opportunities to learn telepsychiatry skills, to work with care managers, to work with a panel of patients, and to develop team-based skills.

2. Residents might want to take ongoing courses and develop a way to be lifelong learners in the area of primary care psychiatry. Programs should develop didactics addressing the issues of CoCM.

3. Primary care partners should provide feedback and evaluation on how the resident is developing skills in primary care psychiatry; the opportunity to receive such feedback should be built into the experiences during residency training.

4. Mentorship and guidance not only from psychiatrists but also from care managers, behavioral health care providers, and primary care clinicians should be obtained.

5. When possible, residents should work with a limited number of primary care clinicians so as to develop communication patterns, to experience warm handoffs, and to recognize practice styles and each other's abilities in order to maximize patient care.

6. The goals of collaborative arrangements should be developed in order to increase trust between providers and primary care physicians who are interested in patients' psychosocial concerns and mental health problems. Patients and families might be asked to complete evaluations on how this system of care is operationalized.

7. Training programs should include and evaluate competencies in team-based care and collaborative care so as to signal proficiencies and career pathways for residents.

8. Technological approaches to care should be included in didactics and clinical experiences. Even though residents themselves might not become experts in all these technologies, at least they will be aware of the panoply of options available to their patients and will be able to have conversations with patients about these offerings.

9. Training should include rotations in facilities providing primary care/ behavioral health integrated care.

10. Residents should apply all the issues regarding split/collaborative treatment discussed in Chapters 5 ("Selection of Medication, Psychotherapy, and Clinicians in Split/Collaborative Treatment") and 6 ("Evaluation and Opening in Split/Collaborative Treatment") to the split/collaborative treatment situation with primary care.

11. Treatment of patients in some resident clinics (or private offices) that are not part of any integrated primary care system may create an even more complicated treatment situation—a "tetradic" configuration involving the patient, resident, therapist, and primary care physician. This configuration provides even more potential for splitting. The risk of adverse outcomes and liability may also increase.

12. Ideas about teaching residents how to talk to patients about medications (Kavanagh et al. 2017) and how to discuss the issues of split/collaborative treatment and a triadic alliance (Mintz 2005) could be applied and expanded into teaching residents to collaborate or consult with primary care physicians.

Competency

Psychiatry residents should become familiar with various technologies (e.g., telepsychiatry) through which they can consult with the primary care team.

Competency

Psychiatry residents should be able to provide consultation regarding patients with a comorbid severe mental disorder and physical illness, such as diabetes mellitus or hypertension.

Competency

Residents should be able to discuss with the primary care physician issues such as the goals and expected outcome of psychiatric consultation/treatment, difficulties in communication, the management of side effects, the fostering of adherence, the role of psychotherapy, and the joint effort to promote a healthy lifestyle for the patient.

Recommendations in Split/Collaborative Treatment in Primary Care

1. When the primary care physician is caring for a patient in a split/collaborative arrangement, there should be an understanding of what is being treated—for example, the patient, the family caring for a patient, the chronic medical condition, or the associated emotional issues (Riba 2001).
2. The primary care physician should be attentive to what is going on in the relationship between himself or herself and the patient, the patient and the mental health clinician, and himself or herself and the mental health clinician (Riba 2001). Ideally, more frequent meetings, telephone calls, or care manager calls should be scheduled.
3. Because psychotropic medications can almost never address all the patient's psychosocial problems, there must be target symptoms (e.g., sleep, appetite, depressed mood, energy) that are addressed with medication; other symptoms may be addressed with psychotherapy or additional forms of treatment (Riba 2001).
4. If the patient is seeing a resident or therapist, the primary care physician and resident or therapist should arrange to discuss their mutual patient and their treatment plans and let the patient know about these discussions (Riba 2001). Furthermore, the clinicians should determine how communication will be conducted in the future (e.g., electronic record, telephone calls).
5. The primary care physician and resident or therapist should discuss diagnostic impressions so that there is agreement and understanding about what is being treated (Riba 2001).
6. It is helpful for the resident and/or therapist and primary care physician to discuss their professional backgrounds and beliefs regarding how they view the relative importance of psychotherapy and pharmacotherapy (Riba 2001).
7. It should be made clear to the patient what type of symptoms are most appropriate to bring to the clinicians' attentions. In addition, confidentiality of issues should be discussed by the primary care physician with the patient. Together, they should determine what medical and psychiatric issues the primary care physician can discuss with the resident, the therapist, family members, and others (Riba 2001).
8. Each clinician and the patient should know when the other clinicians are on vacation and who will cover for the patient regarding mental health problems (Riba 2001).
9. If there is a significant dynamic issue (e.g., suicidal thoughts or intent), the clinicians should determine that they will contact one another and collaboratively address the problem (Riba 2001).

Conclusion

As noted by Unützer (2015, p. 26), "The field of integrated care is young, and there is still much work to do if we want to better leverage the skills of psychiatrists to reach the millions of individuals who are suffering from untreated mental health and substance use problems each year. New partnerships and new technologies are offering us important opportunities to reach this ambitious goal." The Collaborative Care Model should be gradually incorporated into psychiatry residency education, especially during consultation/liaison rotations and psychosomatic medicine fellowships. Novel models of teaching residents how to collaborate with primary care physicians and how to become more fully involved with integrated health care systems are greatly needed.

References

Brown JB, Weston WW: A survey of residency-trained family physicians and their referral of psychosocial problems. Fam Med 24(3):193–196, 1992 1577211

Gitlin MJ, Miklowitz DJ: Split treatment: recommendations for optimal use in the care of psychiatric patients. Ann Clin Psychiatry 28(2):132–137, 2016 27285393

Huffman JC, Niazi SK, Rundell JR, et al: Essential articles on collaborative care models for the treatment of psychiatric disorders in medical settings: a publication by the academy of psychosomatic medicine research and evidence-based practice committee. Psychosomatics 55(2):109–122, 2014 24370112

Katon WJ, Lin EH, Von Korff M, et al: Collaborative care for patients with depression and chronic illnesses. N Engl J Med 363(27):2611–2620, 2010a 21190455

Katon WJ, Unützer J, Wells K, et al: Collaborative depression care: history, evolution and ways to enhance dissemination and sustainability. Gen Hosp Psychiatry 32(5): 456–464, 2010b 20851265

Kavanagh EP, Cahill J, Arbuckle MR, et al: Psychopharmacology prescribing workshops: a novel method for teaching psychiatry residents how to talk to patients about medications. Acad Psychiatry 41(4):491–496, 2017 28194682

Knickman J, Krishnan R, Pincus H: Improving access to effective care for people with mental health and substance use disorders. JAMA 316(16):1647–1648, 2016 27668948

Melek SP, Norris DT, Paulus J: Economic Impact of Integrated Medical-Behavioral Healthcare: Implications for Psychiatry. Denver, CO, Milliman, April 2014

Mintz DL: Teaching the prescriber's role: the psychology of psychopharmacology. Acad Psychiatry 29(2):187–194, 2005 15937266

Ratzliff A, Unützer J: Applying the integrated care approach: practical skills for the psychiatric consultant. American Psychiatric Association Course for District Branches (jointly sponsored by the APA and SAMHSA), July 8, 2016

Ratzliff A, Norfleet K, Chan YF, et al: Perceived educational need of the integrated care psychiatric consultant. Acad Psychiatry 39(4):448–456, 2015 26122347

Reiss-Brennan B, Brunisholz KD, Dredge C, et al: Association of integrated team-based care with health care quality, utilization, and cost. JAMA 316(8):826–834, 2016 27552616

Riba MB: Collaborative treatment for psychiatric patients in the primary care setting: challenges for the doctor-patient relationship. Prim Psychiatry 44:29–31, 2001

Schwenk TL: Integrated behavioral and primary care: what is the real cost? JAMA 316(8):822–823, 2016 27552614

Unützer J: Improving the reach and effectiveness of integrated care. Psychiatr News, November 3, 2015. Available at: http://psychnews.psychiatryonline.org/doi/full/10.1176/appi.pn.2015.11a19. Accessed May 25, 2017.

Valenstein M: Primary care physicians and mental health professionals: models for collaboration, in Psychopharmacology and Psychotherapy: A Collaborative Approach. Edited by Riba MB, Balon R. Washington, DC, American Psychiatric Press, 1999, pp 325–352

Voelker R: Communication gaps hinder full recovery from depression. JAMA 285(11): 1431–1433, 2001 11255402

Wiles N, Thomas L, Abel A, et al: Cognitive behavioural therapy as an adjunct to pharmacotherapy for primary care based patients with treatment resistant depression: results of the CoBalT randomised controlled trial. Lancet 381(9864):375–384, 2013 23219570

Appendix

Review Questions on Competencies Related to Integrated and Split/Collaborative Care

Section 1: Multiple Choice

Choose the *single best answer* for questions 1–7.

A. Integrated care.
B. Split/collaborative care.
C. Both.
D. Neither.

_____ 1. May occur when a patient seeks mental health care for the first time.

_____ 2. Characterized by the psychiatrist providing both pharmacotherapy and psychotherapy.

_____ 3. Characterized by increased prevalence in clinical settings in the United States.

_____ 4. Characterized by a prescribing psychiatrist working closely with another clinician who provides psychotherapy.

_____ 5. Involves attention to fostering a therapeutic alliance with the patient.

_____ 6. Is always limited to 6 months.

_____ 7. Does not require an initial history and mental status examination.

Choose the *single best answer* for questions 8–9.

8. Which of the following statements is correct regarding integrated care or split/collaborative care and the Accreditation Council for Graduate Medical Education's core competency areas for residents?

    A. Six core competencies have direct relevance to integrated care.

    B. No core competencies have direct relevance to integrated care.

    C. Evidence-based assessments have been firmly established regarding integrated care.

    D. Evidence-based assessments have been firmly established regarding split/collaborative care.

9. Which of the following statements is correct regarding integrated care or split/collaborative care with respect to termination of treatment?

    A. Termination of care amounts to patient abandonment and should not occur once a therapeutic relationship is established.

    B. Termination of care amounts to patient abandonment and should not occur once a patient has paid for services.

    C. Termination of care is not the equivalent of patient abandonment if it is initiated by the clinician.

    D. Termination of care is not the equivalent of patient abandonment if it is initiated by the patient.

    E. Termination of care is not the equivalent of patient abandonment if it is in the patient's interests and the mutual decision of the patient and the clinician.

Choose the *single best answer* for questions 10–18.

    A. Integrated care.

    B. Split/collaborative care.

    C. Both.

    D. Neither.

_____ 10. Family members are intentionally excluded in this model of care.

_____ 11. Informed consent is not necessary in this model of care.

_____ 12. Informed consent is necessary in this model of care.

_____ 13. Confidentiality safeguards exist to protect patient information in this model of care.

_____ 14. Frequent communication among clinicians is especially important in this model of care for patients with a personality disorder.

_____ 15. Framing the initial evaluation of a patient as a "consultation" may be helpful in managing expectations around medication.

_____ 16. Treatment should be attuned to diagnostic issues as well as stressors in the patient's life.

_____ 17. Countertransference issues do not arise in this model of care.

_____ 18. A thorough biopsychosocial formulation is especially important in this model of care.

Choose the *single best answer* for questions 19–21.

19. Approximately what percentage of adults in the United States experienced some form of mental disorder in 2014?

   A. 0–5%.
   B. 15%–20%.
   C. 40%–45%.
   D. 55%–60%.
   E. 75%–80%.

20. Which of the following is a potential pitfall in split/collaborative care?

   A. Poorly defined roles.
   B. Poor communication.
   C. Overvaluation of medication.
   D. Undervaluation of medication.
   E. All of the above.

21. One-on-one supervision of residents engaged in split/collaborative care should *not* include which of the following elements?

   A. Frequent discussion of the roles of different clinicians on the treatment team.
   B. Frequent discussion of medication selection and dosing.
   C. Frequent discussion of problematic behavior of a fellow trainee.
   D. Frequent discussion of problematic behavior of the patient.
   E. Frequent discussion of countertransferential issues.

Choose the *single best answer* for questions 22–25.

    A. Integrated care.

    B. Split/collaborative care.

    C. Both.

    D. Neither.

_____ 22. Insurers may not provide payment or reimbursement for this model of care.

_____ 23. Patients are never required to pay out of pocket expenses for this model of care.

_____ 24. This model of care may be appropriate for older adults with depression.

_____ 25. This model of care may be appropriate for adults with substance use disorders.

Choose the *single best answer* for questions 26–28.

26. What psychotherapeutic modality has been shown to provide additional benefit to medication in the treatment of major depression?

    A. Cognitive-behavioral therapy.

    B. Psychodynamic psychotherapy.

    C. Both of the above.

    D. None of the above.

27. What moderating factors may negatively impact treatment of depression in both integrated and split/collaborative care arrangements?

    A. Personality disorders.

    B. Past trauma.

    C. Both of the above.

    D. None of the above.

28. Which of the following professionals prescribe the greatest number of psychotropic medications in the United States?

    A. Primary care physicians.

    B. Psychiatrists.

    C. Psychologists.

Section 2: Questions for Discussion and Self-Reflection

Discuss questions 1–12 with a mentor or colleague:

1. What experiences have you had with split/collaborative care in your training?

2. What experiences have you had with integrative care in your training?

3. What special challenges does split/collaborative care pose for psychiatrists when compared with integrated care?

4. What aspects of split/collaborative care fit well in primary care settings? In community-based mental health settings? In hospital settings?

5. How does transference differ in the context of split/collaborative care when compared with long-term individual psychotherapy?

6. What are best practices in establishing appropriate communication patterns and confidentiality boundaries in split/collaborative care models?

7. How should residents approach supervision to build their knowledge and develop their skills and professional attitudes when learning about integrated care?

8. How does a clinician approach termination of care with the patient and with colleagues on the clinical care team in the context of integrated care or split/collaborative care?

9. How do integrated care and split/collaborative care relate to the Accreditation Council for Graduate Medical Education (ACGME) core competencies?

10. What aspects of the role of the psychiatrist in integrated care and in split/collaborative care models are more comfortable for the early career psychiatrist? What aspects may be more challenging?

11. How might digital or electronic strategies be used in the context of integrated care or split/collaborative care?

12. What new models of care are evolving to address the needs of the increasing number of individuals with mental health issues? How might these models of care move toward supporting recovery and resilience in individuals with mental health issues?

Section 3: Answers to Multiple-Choice Questions (Section 1)

1. C
2. A
3. C
4. B
5. C
6. D
7. D
8. A
9. E
10. D
11. D
12. C
13. C
14. B
15. C
16. C
17. D
18. C
19. B
20. E
21. C
22. C
23. D
24. C
25. C
26. C
27. C
28. A

Index

*Page numbers printed in **boldface** type refer to tables.*

157